The Essential Intensivist Bronchoscopist

Bronchoscopy in the Intensive Care Unit

Modules I - IV

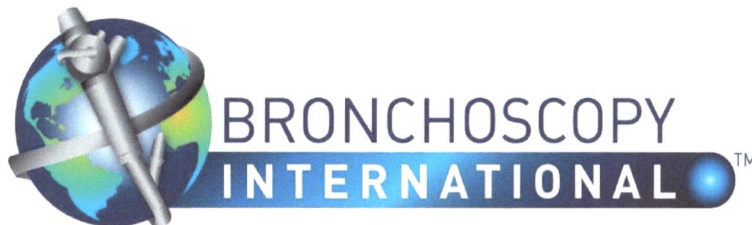

Septimiu Murgu MD, FCCP, Tayfun Caliskan MD, Hugo Oliveira MD, and Henri Colt, MD, FCCP, FAWM

With contributions from Drs. John Mullon, Fabien Maldonado, Shaheen Islam, and Patricia Vujacich

THE ESSENTIAL INTENSIVIST BRONCHOSCOPIST©

rake
press

Laguna Beach, CA

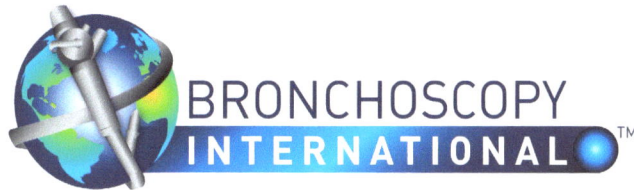

This module was specifically designed for training bronchoscopists working in the intensive care unit. The module and its post-tests, as well as accompanying interactive Powerpoint© presentations are part of a multidimensional curriculum that includes step-by-step hands-on instruction, simulation, instructional videos, patient-based practical approach exercises, and didactic lectures.

This educational program has been designed in collaboration with the following members of the Bronchoscopy International team:

Dr. John Mullon (Rochester, USA)

Dr. Fabien Maldonado (Nashville, USA))

Dr. Shaheen Islam (Columbus, USA)

Dr. Patricia Vujacich (Buenos Aires, Argentina)

Bronchoscopy International, Laguna Beach, CA 92651

Colt Henri G

The Essential Intensivist Bronchoscopist© First Edition, 2017

From, The Essential Bronchoscopist Series™

Title 1: The Essential Intensivist Bronchoscopist; Pulmonary diseases; Thoracic medicine

ISBN-13: 9780984834754

1. The Essential Flexible Bronchoscopist©
2. The Essential EBUS Bronchoscopist©
3. The Essential cTBNA Bronchoscopist©
4. The Essential Intensivist Bronchoscopist©
5. The Essential Interventional Bronchoscopist
6. The Essentials of Bronchoscopy Education©

Manufactured in the United States of America

1 2 3 4 5 6 7 8 9 10

rake
press

FIRST EDITION

The Essential Intensivist Bronchoscopist

Bronchoscopy in the Intensive Care Unit

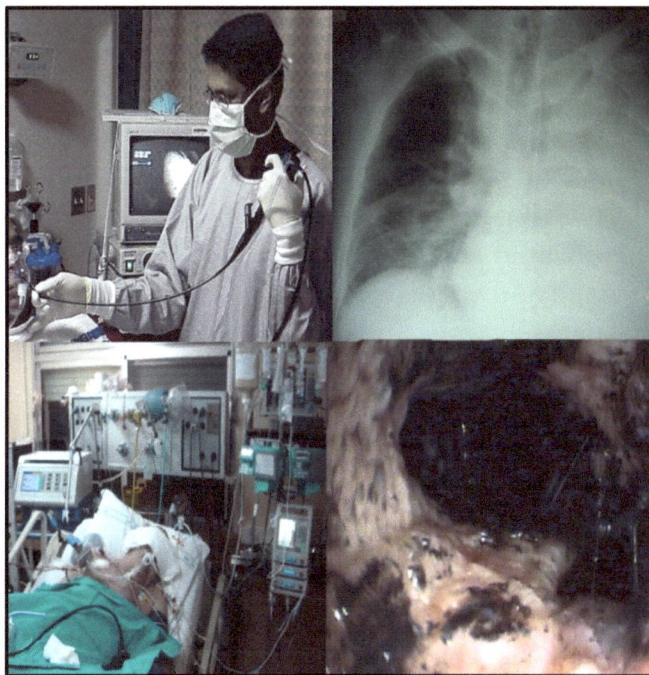

Septimiu Murgu MD, FCCP, Tayfun Caliskan MD, Hugo Oliveira MD, and Henri Colt, MD, FCCP, FAWM

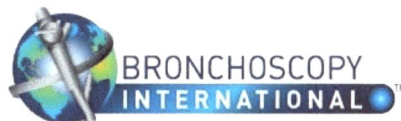

BRONCHOSCOPY INTERNATIONAL™

THE ESSENTIAL BRONCHOSCOPIST™ SERIES

Funding statement

Funding for The Essential Intensivist Bronchoscopist© is a result of collaborative work among members of Bronchoscopy International. No corporate support was either solicited or received for this work.

Acknowledgements

We thank all contributors to the art and science of bronchoscopy in the intensive care unit, and who promote the use of this essential minimally invasive procedure around the world. Particular thanks to Drs. John Mullen, Patricia Vujacich, Rosa Cordovilla, Grigoris Stratakos, Nikos Koufos, Javier Flandes, Maria Simon , Zsolt Papai, Lorenzo Corbetta, Eric Edell, Ales Rozman, Mihai Olteanu, Pedro Mantilla, Domingo Perez, Elizabeth Becerra, Pedro Grynblat, Artemio Garcia, Silvia Quadrelli, Enrique Cases, Jonathan Williamson, David Fielding, Hideo Saka, Eduardo Quintana, Pyng Lee, Omer Elhag, and to the dozens of physicians who promote Bronchoscopy International's philosophy of a medical education without borders.

TABLE OF CONTENTS

Bronchoscopy in the Intensive Care Unit

§

MODULE I

THIRTY MULTIPLE CHOICE QUESTION/ANSWER SETS

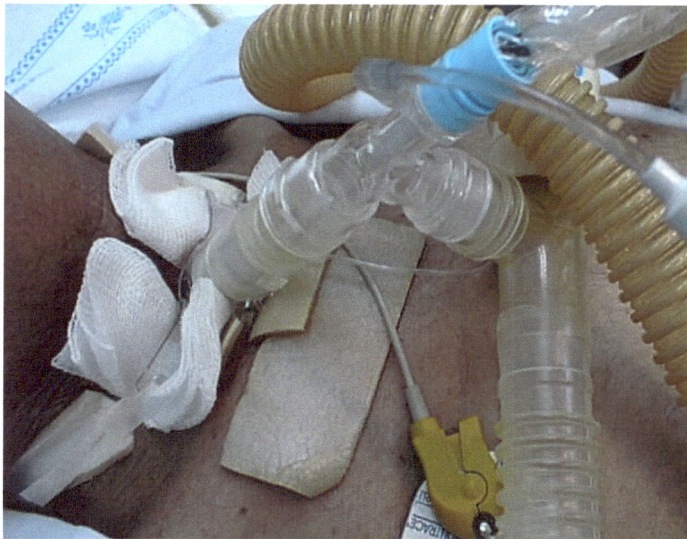

The Essential Intensivist Bronchoscopist©

The Essential Intensivist Bronchoscopist MODULE I

LEARNING OBJECTIVES

After completing this module the reader should be able to:

1. Outline at least three indications and contraindications for performing percutaneous dilatational tracheostomy (PDT).
2. Enumerate at least three advantages and disadvantages of PDT as compared with an open surgical technique.
3. List at least five short and long-term tracheostomy-related complications.
4. Describe step-by-step performance of bronchoscopy-guided PDT.
5. Describe at least three bronchoscopic treatment modalities for critically ill patients with barotrauma or persistent pneumothorax.
6. Identify at least five indications for bronchoscopic intervention in patients with critical central airway obstruction.

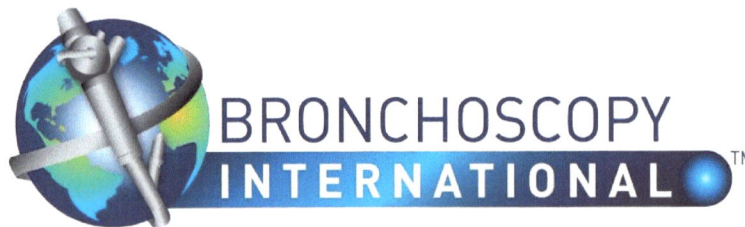

BRONCHOSCOPY INTERNATIONAL™

Question I.1 Which of the following statements about early tracheotomy (performed within ten days after laryngeal endotracheal intubation) is likely <u>true</u>?

A. Early tracheotomy (after 6-8 days of translaryngeal intubation) has statistically significant higher incidence of ventilator-associated pneumonia (VAP) than late tracheotomy in adult patients (after 13-15 days of laryngeal intubation)
B. Early tracheotomy among long-term, mechanically ventilated patients results in a shorter length of stay in the intensive care unit.
C. Early tracheotomy results in lower mortality versus late or no tracheotomy in patients requiring mechanical ventilation.
D. Early tracheotomy (performed within one week of laryngeal intubation) has a lower incidence of pneumonia than late tracheotomy or no tracheotomy in critically ill, mechanically ventilated patients.

Answer I.1:   D

Results comparing early and late tracheotomy in critically ill patients are mixed. In at least one randomized study, there was no difference in the incidence of ventilator-associated pneumonia (VAP) in patients after early tracheotomy (within 6-8 days of translaryngeal intubation) as compared with patients after late tracheotomy (after 13-15 days of laryngeal intubation) (1). At least one meta-analysis found that patients undergoing early tracheotomy (performed within 10 days of intubation) showed no significant difference in clinical outcomes such as reduced length of Intensive Care Unit (ICU) stay for patients on long-term mechanical ventilation (2). In a systematic review and meta-analysis, early tracheostomy was not associated with lower mortality in the ICU when compared with late (more than one week after translaryngeal intubation) or no tracheostomy but was associated with a lower incidence of pneumonia (3).

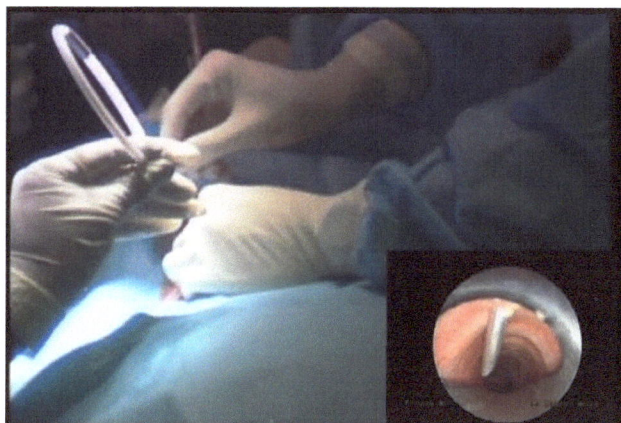

References

1. Terragni PP, Antonelli M, Fumagalli R, Faggiano C, Berardino M, Pallavicini FB, Miletto A, Mangione S, Sinardi AU, Pastorelli M, Vivaldi N, Pasetto A, Della Rocca G, Urbino R, Filippini C, Pagano E, Evangelista A, Ciccone G, Mascia L, Ranieri VM. Early vs late tracheotomy for prevention of pneumonia in mechanically ventilated adult ICU patients: a randomized controlled trial. JAMA 2010; 303(15): 1483-9.
2. Huang H, Li Y, Ariani F, Chen X, Lin J. Timing of tracheostomy in critically ill patients: a meta-analysis. PLoS One 2014; 9(3): e92981.
3. Siempos II, Ntaidou TK, Filippidis FT, Choi AM. Effect of early versus late or no tracheostomy on mortality and pneumonia of critically ill patients receiving mechanical ventilation: a systematic review and meta-analysis. Lancet Respir Med 2015; 3(2): 150-8.

Question I.2: During the informed consent process for a percutaneous tracheostomy, the patient and/or family should be informed that early tracheostomy decreases the risk of mortality at 1 year.

A. True
B. False

Answer I.2: B

A systematic review and meta-analysis assessed the benefit of early (done within 1 week after translaryngeal intubation) versus late (done anytime after the first week of mechanical ventilation) or no tracheostomy on mortality and pneumonia in critically ill patients who needed mechanical ventilation (1). Early tracheostomy was <u>not</u> associated with significantly lower mortality in ICU patients when compared with late or no tracheostomy. Based on these data, at this time, mortality benefit is not an indication for performing early tracheostomy.

Tracheostomy may potentially prevent ventilator-associated pneumonia but not aspiration, or tracheal stenosis. Patient education materials (including a video) should be provided, when feasible.

References

1. Siempos II, Ntaidou TK, Filippidis FT, Choi AM. Effect of early versus late or no tracheostomy on mortality and pneumonia of critically ill patients receiving mechanical ventilation: a systematic review and meta-analysis. Lancet Respir Med 2015; 3(2): 150-8.

Question I.3: Which of the following findings is an absolute contraindication to percutaneous dilatational tracheostomy (PDT)?

A. Limited cervical spine of motion
B. Morbid obesity with BMI>40
C. Site infection

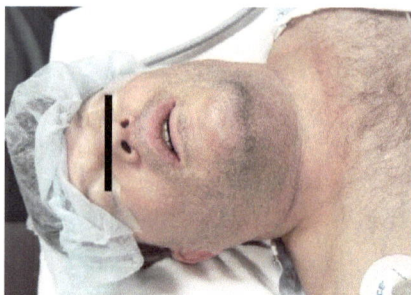

Answer I.3:   C

The only accepted absolute contraindications of the PDT in adults are site infection and uncorrectable coagulopathy. Morbid obesity was considered a relative contraindication however, recent data show that PDT can be performed safely in morbid obesity (2, 3). Similarly, although coagulopathy was described as a relative contraindication, recent literature suggests otherwise (4,5) these days. Other relative contraindications of PDT include high positive end-expiratory pressure (PEEP) or FiO2, limited cervical spine motion, increased intracranial pressure (ICP), hemodynamic instability, re-do tracheotomy, emergent, hemodynamic instability. Anatomic factors considered relative contraindications include: tumor, goiter, unpalpable cricoid cartilage, and tracheomalacia.

References

1. Abouzgheib W, Meena N, Jagtap P, Schorr C, Boujaoude Z, Bartter T. Percutaneous dilatational tracheostomy in patients receiving antiplatelet therapy: is it safe? J Bronchology Interv Pulmonol 2013; 20(4): 322-5.
2. McCague A1, Aljanabi H, Wong DT. Safety analysis of percutaneous dilational tracheostomies with bronchoscopy in the obese patient. Laryngoscope. 2012 May;122(5):1031-4
3. Heyrosa MG, Melniczek DM, Rovito P, Nicholas GG. Percutaneous tracheostomy: a safe procedure in the morbidly obese. J Am Coll Surg. 2006 Apr;202(4):618-22.
4. Pandian V1, Vaswani RS, Mirski MA, Haut E, Gupta S, Bhatti NI. Safety of percutaneous dilational tracheostomy in coagulopathic patients. Ear Nose Throat J. 2010 Aug;89(8):387-95.
5. Takahashi M, Itagaki S, Laskaris J, Filsoufi F, Reddy RC. Percutaneous tracheostomy can be safely performed in patients with uncorrected coagulopathy after cardiothoracic surgery. Innovations (Phila). 2014 Jan-Feb;9(1):22-6.

Question I.4: A patient requiring invasive mechanical ventilation with an endotracheal tube undergoes tracheostomy with a tube of the same diameter. This will reduce airway resistance, work of breathing, and peak airway pressures.

A. True
B. False

Answer I.4. A

Although the small radius of tracheostomy tubes may increase the turbulence of the airflow, their short length compensates for the turbulence. For example, an 8.5 endotracheal tube has a five-fold greater resistance than a comparable tracheostomy tube (1,2). A study of tracheotomy for repeated extubation failure in 20 ventilator-dependent patients noted an improvement in work of breathing (8.9 ± 2.9 vs 6.6 ± 1.4 J/min, respectively; p< 0.04). The beneficial effects were magnified, however, as the respiratory rate increased (3). Peak inspiratory pressure is also decreased after a tracheotomy is performed when compared with the pressures measured through the endotracheal tubes (pre 33.4 ± 11.8 vs post 28.6 ± 9.2 mm Hg) (4).

References

1. Habib, MP. Physiological implications of artificial airways. Chest 1989;96(1):180-4.
2. Yung, MW, Snowdon, SL. Respiratory resistance of tracheostomy tubes. Arch Otolaryngol 198; 110(9): 591-5.
3. Davis, K, Jr, Campbell, RS, Johannigman, JA, Valente JF, Branson RD. Changes in respiratory mechanics after tracheostomy. Arch Surg 1999; 134(1):59-62.
4. Lin, MC, Huang, CC, Yang, CT, Tsai YH, Tsao TC. Pulmonary mechanics in patients with prolonged mechanical ventilation requiring tracheostomy. Anaesth Intensive Care 1999; 27(6): 581-5.

Question I.5: A patient with severe emphysema may be at higher risk for this complication during percutaneous dilatational tracheostomy (PDT):

A. Tracheal-innominate artery fistula
B. Pneumothorax
C. Tracheal ring fracture

Answer I.5: B

A patient with severe emphysema is at high risk for pneumothorax during PDT due to hyper inflated lungs and potential for lung puncture during the tracheocentesis.

Team experience, therefore, is very important when performing this procedure in patients with severe emphysema and hyper-inflated lungs. Operators should be trained to clearly identify upper airway structures and perform the skin incision, the needle insertion and tracheostomy tube insertion in the middle of the inter-cartilaginous space. This will avoid inadvertent puncture of the adjacent lung or vascular structures.

In addition, operators should be able to rapidly aspirate airway secretions, and be able to intubate over the bronchoscope or insert a chest tube emergently if needed. Anatomic dangers for risks related to the procedure are high riding innominate artery, Superior Vena Cava (SVC) syndrome, tracheal deviation, barrel-shaped chest and hyperinflated lungs.

Question I.6: In optimal anatomical circumstances, which inter-cartilaginous space should be chosen for a percutaneous dilatational tracheostomy (PDT)?

A. Cricoid-1st intercartilaginous space
B. 2nd -3rd intercartilaginous space
C. 4th -5th intercartilaginous space

Answer I.6:   B

Ideally, the puncture site (tracheal entry site) is anterior, midline and in between the 2nd-3rd tracheal rings or 3rd-4th rings; a higher tracheostomy tube placement could result in post tracheostomy stenosis, which will be very difficult to manage especially when involving the subglottic area. A lower placement (4th-5th space) could potentially increase the risk for trachea-innominate fistula especially in those patients with a high riding innominate artery.

For a precise tracheal ring selection, the operators should strive for an optimal patient positioning (i.e. supine with neck hyper-extended); Some operators use one or two rolled towels, pillows or bolster in between the scapulae for this purpose; head of bed can be elevated to 20 degrees to reduce venous engorgement.

Herein we describe our technique for performing the PDT.

We prepare the table (a Mayo stand or an ICU room table), and then the tracheostomy tray is opened: the tracheostomy tube cuff is checked for integrity with 10-20 ml of air, then deflated. The # 26 (for Shiley 6) or # 28 (for Shiley 8) dilators are lubrified and inserted inside the corresponding tracheostomy tube.

The puncture site/ tracheal entry site, as mentioned above, is always anterior, midline, between the 2nd-3rd tracheal rings or 3rd-4th rings; we identify the site by palpation after identifying the thyroid cartilage, the cricoid and the first tracheal ring.

Then the site is prepared in a sterile fashion using chlorhexidine. Local analgesia is provided at the entry site subcutaneously in four quadrants using lidocaine 1% mixed with epinephrine. There are several different techniques for performing percutaneous tracheostomy. What follows is a description of one of these techniques:

Exploratory "tracheocentesis" is then performed using a small -needle (finder needle) at the entry site. Once the small needle is confirmed bronchoscopically in the desired location, the large bore needle or the angiocath available in the kit is inserted adjacent to the small finder needle and then the small needle is removed. Then the guidewire is placed: once the large bore needle is clearly visualized via the bronchoscope, the guidewire is advanced with the tip oriented inferiorly, then once inside the airway, the large bore needle is removed (see figure below).

The skin incision is then made one centimeter above and one below the entry port to the subcutaneous fat; we use the # 11 scalpel available in the kit. One could consider a Bovie (portable electrocautery unit) or using the operating theater's electrocautery system especially for cases where bleeding is expected: coagulopathy, anticoagulants, uremia, hepatic insufficiency.

Subcutaneous and initial inter-cartilaginous space dilation is then done by using a small blue dilator after lubrication. The inter-cartilaginous space is dilated, then the cone dilator is inserted over the stiffening catheter and the guidewire; once inside the airway lumen, and once the thick black line is visualized, the dilator is removed but the guidewire and stiffening catheter are left in place. Then the tracheostomy tube is inserted over the dilator into the tracheal lumen.

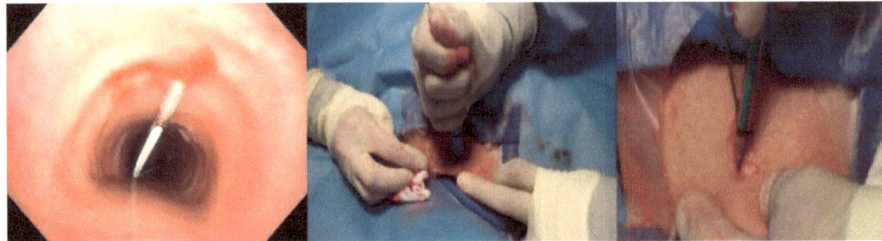

Question I.7: During percutaneous dilatational tracheostomy, after the stoma is dilated, a #8 Shiley tracheostomy tube/28F dilator assembly is advanced over the stiffening catheter but high resistance is encountered. The patient is tachycardic, hypertensive and O2 sat is 90% from 98% on FiO2 of 1. What should be done next?

A.   Use more firm pressure and push the tracheostomy tube in the airway as this is now an emergency
B.   Switch to a smaller size (# 6) Shiley tracheostomy tube and insert it over the bronchoscope
C.   Remove the tracheostomy/dilator assembly and assure there is no gap between the tip of the tracheostomy tube and the dilator

Answer I.7:   C

Repositioning the dilator to close the gap is the most optimal step. Soft tissue/cartilage can be caught in the gap and any force will break the cartilage, causing stomal strictures. Once the gap is closed, the tracheostomy tube and its indwelling dilator can be advanced over the guidewire and stiffening catheter. Once the cuff is completely inside the airway and confirmed by bronchoscopy, the guidewire, the stiffening catheter and the dilator are removed en-block. The inner cannula is placed inside the tracheostomy tube, the cuff is inflated and ventilation is begun via the tracheostomy tube (1).

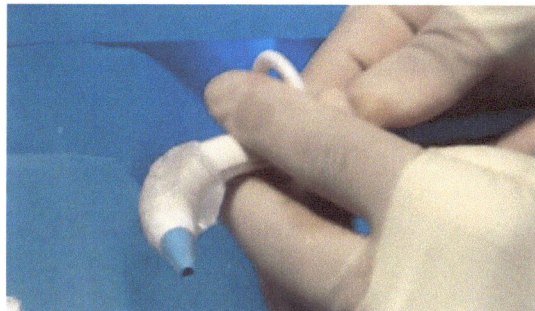

References

1. Heffner JE, Miller KS, Sahn SA. Tracheostomy in the intensive care unit. Part 1: Indications, technique, management. Chest 1986; 90(2):269-74.

Question I.8: A percutaneous dilatational tracheostomy (PDT) is performed in an obese patient. A 6. 0 Shiley tracheostomy tube is inserted. Bronchoscopy shows the cuff fits well inside the trachea with the flange of the tracheostomy tube at the skin. Once the patient wakes up, an air leak is heard despite inflating the cuff. The tidal volumes are low and patient shows signs of distress (tachypnea, tachycardia, and hypertension). What should be done next?

A.   Use more air to overinflate the cuff of the indwelling tracheostomy tube
B.   Exchange the # 6 to an extra-long or larger size tracheostomy tube
C.   Increase sedation while patient is on positive pressure ventilation

Answer I.8:   B

In this case, it appears that the initial tube selection was too short as the patient had a leak in spite of correct positioning and cuff being properly inflated. After placemen, the tracheostomy tube likely was retracted outward and the cuff of the tube is likely partially in the stoma, rather than in the trachea. An extended length tracheostomy tube (E.g. Shiley XLT proximal) will accommodate the increased skin to trachea distance in this obese patient.

Tracheostomy tubes are available in a variety of sizes and styles from several manufacturers. The inner diameter, outer diameter, and any other distinguishing characteristics (percutaneous, extra length, fenestrated) are marked on the flange of the tube as a guide to the clinician (1).

The most commonly used tracheostomy tubes are made from polyvinyl chloride (PVC), silicone, or polyurethane. When selecting a tracheostomy tube, the inner diameter, outer diameter, and length must be considered. If the inner diameter is too small, it will increase the resistance through the tube and make airway clearance more difficult.

A smaller inner diameter tube also has a smaller outer diameter, which may increase the cuff pressure required to create a seal in the trachea. If the outer diameter is too large, however, the leak with the cuff deflated will be decreased, and this will affect the ability to use the upper airway with cuff deflation for speech. A tube with a larger outer diameter will also be more difficult to pass through the stoma. A 10-mm outer diameter tube is usually appropriate for adult women, and an 11-mm outer diameter tube is usually appropriate for adult men as an initial tracheostomy tube size.

References

1. Hess DR, Altobelli NP. Tracheostomy tubes. Respir Care 2014; 59(6): 956-71; discussion 971-3.

Question I.9: During percutaneous dilatational tracheostomy, the tracheostomy tube is placed, ventilation is switched from the endotracheal tube to the tracheostomy tube, and the cuff of the tracheostomy is inflated. What is the next step?

A. The procedure is completed. Educate the nurses/housestaff/family on tracheostomy care
B. Remove the ETT and confirm tracheostomy tube position via bronchoscopy
C. Measure the pressure in the tracheostomy cuff to assure it is < 25 mm Hg

Answer I.9:   B

     After the cuff of the tracheostomy is inflated, the ETT is removed and the tracheostomy tube's exact position should be confirmed via bronchoscopy. The larynx is examined during extubation to document airway findings and measure distance from the cords. The swivel adaptor is connected to the tracheostomy tube, and bronchoscopy is performed to clean the airway from hemorrhagic secretions and measure the distance from the carina to the tip of the tracheostomy tube.

     To secure the tracheostomy tube, four stitches are usually placed over the tracheostomy flange. A tracheostomy tube tie is used as well around the neck allowing room for two fingers between the tie and the neck. Education of the nursing staff is necessary regarding tracheostomy tube position, dressing change and tracheostomy tube change.

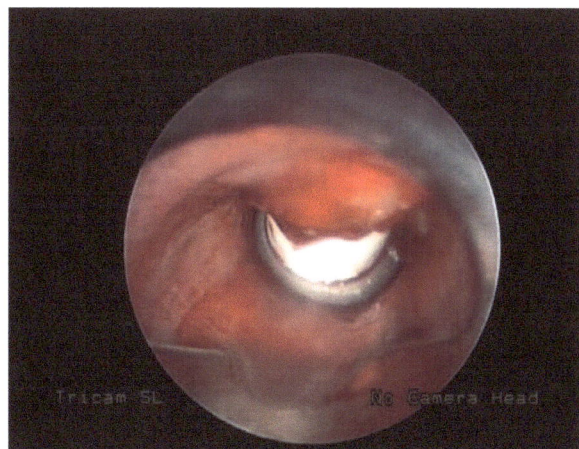

Question I.10: Ciaglia Blue Rhino® G2, Ciaglia Blue Dolphin®, Portex® Blue Line Ultra® Tracheostomy Tube Kit are commonly used percutaneous dilatational tracheostomy (PDT) kits used in the United States. Compared with the Blue Rhino, the Blue Dolphin results in:

A. Less difficulty in passing the tracheostomy tube
B. Less procedure-related airway bleeding
C. Takes longer to place

Answer I.10:   C

Percutaneous dilatational tracheostomy (PDT) is a common procedure in intensive care units and the identification of the best technique is very important. Balloon dilatational tracheostomy using the Ciaglia Blue Dolphin device has been introduced as a modification of the Ciaglia technique. The Ciaglia Blue Dolphin uses an inflatable balloon dilation system instead of the single-step cone dilator.

In one study, the new Dolphin system was compared with the single-step dilatational tracheostomy (Ciaglia Blue Rhino) in intensive care unit (ICU) patients (1). Median procedure length (minutes between tracheal puncture and tracheostomy tube placement) was significantly shorter in the Rhino group than in the Dolphin group. The investigators found minimal bleeding, described either as 'oozing' or as tracheal wall stained with blood at bronchoscopy six hours later, with a higher percentage in the Dolphin group. The study concluded that the Ciaglia Blue Dolphin technique was a viable option in ICU patients, although their findings encouraged the use of Ciaglia Blue Rhino technique because it had a shorter execution time.

A systematic review and meta-analysis of randomized studies comparing different PDT techniques (Multiple dilators, single-step dilatation, guide wire dilating forceps, rotational dilation, retrograde tracheostomy, and balloon dilation techniques) in critically ill adults was performed to investigate if one technique was superior to the others with regard to major and minor intraprocedural complications (2). The different techniques and devices were equivalent, with the exception of:

• Retrograde tracheostomy, which was associated with more severe complications and more frequent need for conversion to other techniques when compared with guide wire dilating forceps and single-step dilatation techniques, and

• Single-step dilatation technique was associated with fewer failures than rotational dilation, and fewer mild complications in comparison with balloon dilation and guide wire dilating forceps.

The authors of this study concluded that single-step dilatation technique was the most reliable from among six different techniques in terms of safety and success rate.

References

1. Cianchi G, Zagli G, Bonizzoli M, Batacchi S, Cammelli R, Biondi S, Spina R, Peris A. Comparison between single-step and balloon dilatational tracheostomy in intensive care unit: a single-center, randomized controlled study. Br J Anaesth 2010; 104(6): 728-32.
2. Cabrini L, Monti G, Landoni G, Biondi-Zoccai G, Boroli F, Mamo D, Plumari VP, Colombo S, Zangrillo A. Percutaneous tracheostomy, a systematic review. Acta Anaesthesiol Scand 2012; 56(3): 270-81.

Question I.11: Results of studies and meta-analysis suggest that compared with the surgical tracheostomy, the percutaneous dilatational technique results in higher rates of:

A.   Bleeding
B.   Mortality
C.   Wound infection
D.   Highly located stenosis

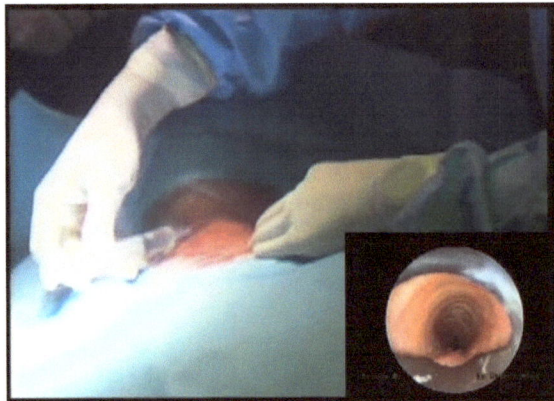

Answer I.11:   D

Elective percutaneous dilatational tracheostomy (PDT) and surgical tracheostomy (ST) in adult critically ill patients with regards to major short and long-term outcomes were compared in a systematic review and meta-analysis (1). PDT reduced the overall incidence of wound infection and further reduced clinical relevant bleeding and mortality when compared with ST performed in the operating room. It was concluded that PDT, performed in the ICU, should be considered the procedure of choice for performing elective tracheostomies in critically ill adult patients.

Because clinically relevant stomal post-tracheostomy stenosis depends mainly on the puncture site and tracheal fractures during PDT, adequate endoscopic guidance during PDT is important (2).

Subjective voice changes and tracheal abnormalities are common after endotracheal intubation followed by PDT.

Long-term follow-up of critically ill patients identified a 31% rate of tracheal stenosis after PDT (defined as more than 10% narrowing). Symptomatic stenosis manifested by subjective respiratory symptoms after decannulation is found in 6% of the patients (3). In another study, subclinical tracheal stenosis was found in about 40% of patients following PDT (4).

References

1. Delaney A, Bagshaw SM, Nalos M. Percutaneous dilatational tracheostomy versus surgical tracheostomy in critically ill patients: a systematic review and meta-analysis. Crit Care 2006; 10(2): R55.
2. Dollner R, Verch M, Schweiger P, Graf B, Wallner F. Long-term outcome after Griggs tracheostomy. J Otolaryngol 2002; 31(6): 386-9.
3. Norwood S, Vallina VL, Short K, Saigusa M, Fernandez LG, McLarty JW. Incidence of tracheal stenosis and other late complications after percutaneous tracheostomy. Ann Surg 2000; 232(2): 233-41.
4. Walz MK, Peitgen K, Thürauf N, Trost HA, Wolfhard U, Sander A, Ahmadi C, Eigler FW. Percutaneous dilatational tracheostomy--early results and long-term outcome of 326 critically ill patients. Intensive Care Med 1998; 24(7): 685-90.

Question I.12: The rate of false lumen creation is higher with the open surgical technique than with the percutaneous dilatational tracheostomy (PDT).

A. True
B. False

Answer I.12:   B

Multiple studies have been performed to characterize differences in complications and cost-effectiveness of PDT and surgical tracheostomy (ST). In a meta-analysis, there were significantly fewer complications in the PDT group with respect to wound infection and unfavorable scarring (1). There was no statistically significant difference between PDT and ST for complications of false passage, minor hemorrhage, major hemorrhage, subglottic stenosis, death, and overall complications. However, overall complication rates trended toward favoring the percutaneous technique. PDT case length was shorter overall by 4.6 minutes, and costs were reduced by approximately $456 USD as compared with surgical tracheostomy.

The choice between PDT and ST was evaluated using the quality of evidence in 37 published articles comparing the two methods (2). From these studies, 4 were meta-analyses, 17 were randomized controlled trials, 13 comparative studies, 2 prospective nonrandomized studies and 1 prospective randomized. Taking into account the complication rate from these studies, 7 are in favor of PDT and 3 in favor of ST. Given the low level of evidence, however, the authors concluded that any claims by clinicians in favor of a particular treatment are still debatable.

References

1. Higgins KM, Punthakee X. Meta-analysis comparison of open versus percutaneous tracheostomy. Laryngoscope 2007; 117(3): 447-54.
2. Pappas S, Maragoudakis P, Vlastarakos P, Assimakopoulos D, Mandrali T, Kandiloros D, Nikolopoulos TP. Surgical versus percutaneous tracheostomy: an evidence-based approach. Eur Arch Otorhinolaryngol 2011; 268(3): 323-30.

Question I.13: A surgical approach is favored over percutaneous dilatational tracheostomy (PDT) when:

A.   Vascular structures are palpated over the planned tracheal site
B.   The patient is morbidly obese with a BMI>40
C.   There is evidence of infection at the site of planned tracheostomy
D.   There is a history of previous surgical tracheostomy

Answer I.13:   A

Complications of PDT are traditionally divided into early and late. Early complications include bleeding, infection, pneumothorax, technical failures and perioperative hypoxia due to tube obstruction or accidental decannulation (1). The major late complications include development of granulation tissue resulting in airway stenosis, failure to decannulate or upper airway obstruction with respiratory failure after decannulation, tracheoesophageal fistula, tracheomalacia, tracheal stenosis and tracheoinnominate artery fistula (TIF).

Most complications of PDT are late complications, mainly airway stenosis and accidental decannulation and to a lesser extent TIF. Bleeding is most common in the early postoperative period. Intraoperative complications of tracheostomy by any technique are rare. Fatal complications of PDT have only been reported in a small number of cases and fatal intraoperative complications of PDT are even less common. Almost all result from vascular injury. Any vascular pulsation palpated over the tracheostomy site mandates preoperative ultrasound or conversion to open surgical tracheostomy.

References
1. Gilbey P. Fatal complications of percutaneous dilatational tracheostomy. Am J Otolaryngol 2012; 33(6): 770-3.

Question I.14: The majority of percutaneous dilatational tracheostomy (PDT) related-fatal complications occur after the first month post procedure.

A.   True
B.   False

Answer I.14:   B

PDT can be associated with major complications, including death. The causes of lethal complications due to PDT were analyzed in a systematic review (1). The incidence of lethal complications was calculated to be 0.17%. The major causes of death were tracheostomy-related hemorrhage in 38% of these patients and airway complications in 29.6% of these patients. In 31% of cases, fatal complications occurred during the procedure and in 49.3% of cases within seven days of the procedure; 73.2% of patients had specific risk factors and 25.4% of patients had more than one risk factor.

According to this analysis, PDT-related death occurs in 1 out of 600 patients receiving a PDT. Careful patient selection, bronchoscopic guidance, and securing the tracheal cannula with sutures are likely to reduce complication rates.

References

1. Simon M, Metschke M, Braune SA, Püschel K, Kluge S. Death after percutaneous dilatational tracheostomy: a systematic review and analysis of risk factors. Crit Care 2013; 17(5): R258.

Question I.15: Accidental decannulation and inability to replace the tracheostomy tube leads to death in percutaneous dilatational tracheostomy (PDT) but not in the surgical tracheostomy (ST) groups.

A.   True
B.   False

Answer I.15:   B

There is an ongoing debate about whether percutaneous dilatational tracheostomy (PDT) is better than ST in regards to safety. The hypothesis that PDT would be superior to ST in regards to efficacy, perioperative and postoperative complications, and long-term (>12 months) follow-up was evaluated in a study (1). Accidental decannulation and inability to replace the tracheotomy tube led to a similar rate of deaths in both STs (N=8) and PDTs (N=9). In addition, no tracheal stenosis was detected at 20 months in either group.

References

1. Silvester W, Goldsmith D, Uchino S, Bellomo R, Knight S, Seevanayagam S, Brazzale D, McMahon M, Buckmaster J, Hart GK, Opdam H, Pierce RJ, Gutteridge GA. Percutaneous versus surgical tracheostomy: A randomized controlled study with long-term follow-up. Crit Care Med 2006; 34(8): 2145-52.

Question I.16: A patient with a tracheostomy performed 3 weeks ago has accidental decannulation while turning in bed. His tracheostomy was performed for a laryngeal tumor and he is currently undergoing external beam radiation therapy. Attempt to re-insert the same tracheostomy tube failed. The patient is in respiratory distress. Which of the following steps is most indicated immediately?

A.   Attempt to insert a smaller size tracheostomy tube
B.   Occlude the tracheostomy stoma and call for help
C.   Administer oxygen both via tracheostomy stoma and face mask
D.   Proceed with oral intubation and summon emergency assistance

Answer I.16:   C

Three weeks after tracheostomy the tracheostomy stoma should have matured and a smaller size tracheostomy tube insertion might be the most appropriate maneuver. Any difficulty encountered while inserting the tube, however, might signal airway obstruction at the stomal level due to tumor, granulation tissue or chondritis/malacia. Oxygen can be administered via the tracheostomy stoma and by facemask. An emergency airway may be obtained by bronchoscopic re-intubation orally with a small size endotracheal tube, or by placing an endotracheal tube through the stoma into the trachea. It would be wrong to occlude the stoma and call for help, because the tracheostomy stoma may represent the patient's sole airway, especially if the suprastomal airway is occluded by laryngeal tumor or radiation-induced swelling.

Question I.17: A percutaneous dilatational tracheostomy (PDT) was performed 6 hours ago. The nurse calls to report bleeding at the stoma site. The dressing is soaked with blood, but there is no obvious bleeding source. What should be done next?

A. Inject lidocaine with epinephrine around the stoma
B. Suspect tracheo-innominate artery fistula and emergent thoracic surgery consultation
C. Order PT, PTT, CBC and a chest radiograph

Answer I.17:　　　　A

If bleeding occurs immediately after the incision is made, electro cauterization and a hemostat may be used. If it occurs after dilation is finished, then operators should promptly insert the tracheostomy tube. If bleeding occurs after the procedure, then lidocaine with epinephrine in the four quadrants can be re-injected. If bleeding recurs or persists, Surgicel should be placed and the stoma will need to be explored either at bedside or in OR to search for a source. In most cases, a slow bleeding vein or capillary oozing is the cause and it can be cauterized or ligated. Tracheo-innominate artery fistula usually occurs after 3-6 weeks of placement and should be considered if there is delayed bleeding and a thoracic/ ENT surgeon should be consulted immediately. In the post-procedure period, the gauze can be removed on day 1. Ventilator tubing should not be "pulling" on the tracheostomy tube. Cuff pressure should be checked daily. Sutures can be removed 7-14 days post-procedure, and at 14-21 days for tracheostomy tube change. Many specialists, however, do not place any sutures after tracheostomy tube placement! If the patient tolerates a tracheostomy tube collar, speech therapy can be consulted for placement of a Passy Muir Valve. A nutritional evaluation may also be warranted.

Question I.18: In surgical tracheostomy, the first tracheostomy tube change is ideally performed by:

A.   A certified critical care nurse
B.   A certified respiratory therapist
C.   An ear nose and throat surgeon
D.   The service that performed the procedure

Answer I.18:   D

The first tracheostomy tube change should be performed by the primary service or their designees. Ideally, two trained caregivers (Respiratory therapist and a registered nurse, for example) should be present during tracheostomy tube changes. In adult patients, a trained therapist will subsequently change the tracheostomy tube once per week following the initial change. Tracheostomy ties and stoma dressings should be changed at least every 48 hours and as needed. Tracheostomy cuffs should be filled with air or sterile water (as ordered). Normal saline is not recommended. During hospitalization, tracheostomy cuff volume should be checked every shift. Routine cuff deflation is not recommended. Faulty cuffs should be reported to the procedural service.

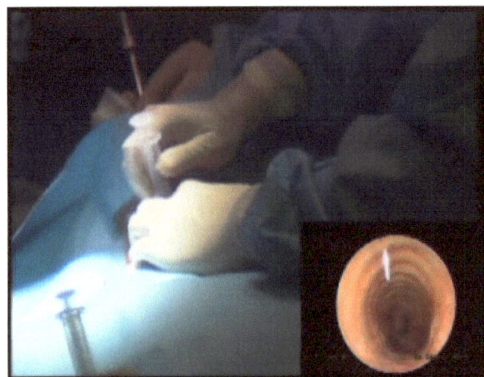

Question 1.19: Prior to performing percutaneous dilatational tracheostomy, it is important to carefully examine results from which of the following?

A. Medication use, renal function and coagulation profile
B. End-tidal CO2 measurements
C. Endotracheal tube cuff pressure measurements

Answer I.19:   A

  The initial evaluation before percutaneous dilatational tracheostomy (PDT) should include three components:
  1) Physical exam: site infection, inability to identify laryngeal/tracheal anatomy (such as in patients with high BMI, thyroid masses), neck immobility (rheumatoid arthritis, cervical spine disease, post radiation) represent contraindications to PDT. Site infection is an absolute contraindication because it can lead to stomal infections and mediastinitis;
  2) Evaluation for co-morbidities such as increased intracranial pressure (ICP), severe chronic obstructive pulmonary disease, hypoxemic respiratory failure with high FiO2 (> 60%) and positive end-expiratory pressure (PEEP) requirements (> 10 cm H_2O). Other contraindications include hemodynamically unstable patient; expected short-term intubation and expected short-term survival;
  3) Presence of a coagulopathy. For example, systemic anticoagulation and potent antiplatelet agents (i.e. clopidogrel) should be held prior to performing the procedure, although there is evidence that PDT can be performed safely on clopidogrel and that aspirin can be continued. Overall, it is warranted to keep the INR< 1.5 and platelets > 50. In end-stage renal disease patients, the procedure should ideally be performed on non-hemodialysis (HD) day or immediately after HD.

References

1. Abouzgheib W, Meena N, Jagtap P, Schorr C, Boujaoude Z, Bartter T. Percutaneous dilatational tracheostomy in patients receiving antiplatelet therapy: is it safe? J Bronchology Interv Pulmonol 2013; 20(4): 322-5.

Question I.20. Patients with severe emphysema have which of the following findings on clinical examination (performed in preparation for percutaneous dilatational tracheostomy)

A. Short laryngeal height (distance between the thyroid cartilage and the sternal notch)
B. Ipsilateral tracheal deviation
C. Increased incidence of prognathia

Answer I.20:　　　　A

   Patients with severe emphysema may have a short laryngeal height (distance between the thyroid cartilage and the sternal notch) and thus the cervical trachea may be surrounded by lung parenchyma bilaterally, thus representing a risk of pneumothorax.
   During the informed consent process, patients and their families should be told of the possible risks of pneumothorax, as well as of other possible procedure-related adverse events such as infection, bleeding, loss of airway (intraoperative or post-op due to tracheostomy tube dislodgment), cartilage fracture, tracheal stenosis, vocal cords dysfunction, dysphagia, aspiration, and loss of voice and these risks should be documented prior to the procedure.

Question I.21. Which of the following statements pertaining to post-tracheotomy stenosis is <u>true</u>?

A. Monitoring intracuff pressures is no longer relevant with the advent of modern tracheotomy tubes.
B. Strictures at the level of the tracheostomy tube cuff can be caused by ischemic mucosal damage.
C. The incidence of stomal strictures has actually increased since the use of high volume-low pressure cuffs.

Answer I.21:   B

Stenoses at the level of the tracheostomy tube cuff are usually caused by ischemic mucosal damage when cuff to tracheal wall tension exceeds mucosa capillary perfusion pressure (usually 20-30 mm Hg) (1). Inflammatory histologic changes occur within 24-48 hours. Incidence has been reduced tenfold after transition to high volume-low pressure cuffs. Intracuff pressures must be closely monitored, maintaining both peak inspiratory and expiratory intracuff pressures below 15 mm Hg (definitely below 25 mm Hg).

Question I.22: Stenosis after percutaneous dilatational tracheostomy occurs most often in which of the following regions?

A. Suprastomal region of the trachea
B. Stomal region of the trachea
C. Subglottic region of the trachea
D. At the level of the tracheostomy tube cuff

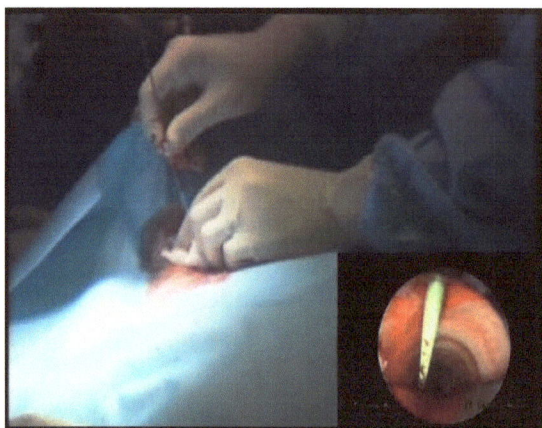

Answer I.22:   C

Tracheostomy-induced tracheal stenosis occurs in 3 regions: in the suprastomal region, at the level of the cuff and at the stomal site. Stenosis caused by percutaneous dilatational tracheostomy (PDT) may occur earlier and is subglottic in nature compared to that caused by surgical tracheostomy.

Surgical correction of stenosis is more difficult in the PDT group due to its presentation in the subglottic area (1). Thus, the tracheal midline should be used during PDT procedure as much as possible. A side-placed tracheostomy tube puts tension on the tracheal wall and may cause skin necrosis and cartilage damage. If the skin incision is too small, and the tracheostomy tube becomes stuck during insertion, one should gently pull the tube back but leave the guidewire and the catheter inside the tracheal lumen, and enlarge the incision to the subcutaneous tissue; this will avoid exerting excess tension on the tracheal wall during dilation.

References

1. Raghuraman G, Rajan S, Marzouk JK, Mullhi D, Smith FG. Is tracheal stenosis caused by percutaneous tracheostomy different from that by surgical tracheostomy? Chest 2005; 127(3): 879-85.

Question I.23: You are called to assist a thoracic surgeon perform percutaneous tracheostomy. After inserting the flexible bronchoscope, you notice the abnormality shown in the image below. What is the significance of this abnormality?

A. Generally seen in pigs, dogs, and camels.
B. Accessory bronchus that can be found as high as 6 centimeters above the carina, and thus be obstructed in case of a long tracheotomy tube or endotracheal tube.
C. Usually asymptomatic, but often a cause for recurrent bronchitis, hemoptysis, or pneumonia.

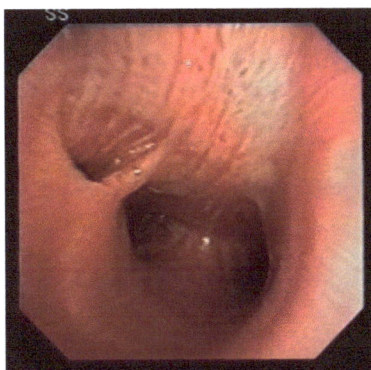

Answer 1.23:   B

A tracheal bronchus is an anatomic variant where an accessory bronchus originates directly from the trachea and is directed to the upper lobe territory. It is often called a pig bronchus, although this nomenclature is usually reserved for cases where the entire upper lobe (usually right side) is supplied by this bronchus. A tracheal bronchus is a normal finding in sheep, pigs, goats, and giraffes. In humans, the prevalence is 0.1-2% on the right side and 0.3-1% on the left. When a true supernumerary bronchus originates from the left or right main bronchus, it is often referred to as a cardiac bronchus (frequency 0.3%).

If the anatomical right upper lobe bifurcates, the tracheal bronchus is described as displaced. If the right upper lobe trifurcates, the tracheal bronchus is described as supernumerary (1). Normal tracheobronchial development occurs 24–26 days as a median bulge of the ventral wall of the pharynx developing at the caudal end of the laryngotracheal groove. At 26–28 days, this bulge gives rise to right and left lung buds, and development, including the formation of segmental bronchi, is usually complete by day 36.   Several hypotheses are offered to explain the formation of accessory bronchi, including the reduction theory (shrinkage of primitive components), selection theory (local disturbances of morphogenesis), and migration theory (an outgrowth of derivative branches) (2).

The tracheal bronchus may be the cause of recurrent bronchitis or pneumonia, especially when the right upper lobe is involved. It should also be suspected in patients with possible right upper lobe cyst on chest radiographs. It has not been associated with an increased frequency of hemoptysis. Although usually located at the level of or within 2 centimeters of the carina, a tracheal bronchus may be found as high as 6 centimeters above the main carina, and thus be easily blocked by a low-lying endotracheal tube or long tracheotomy tube.

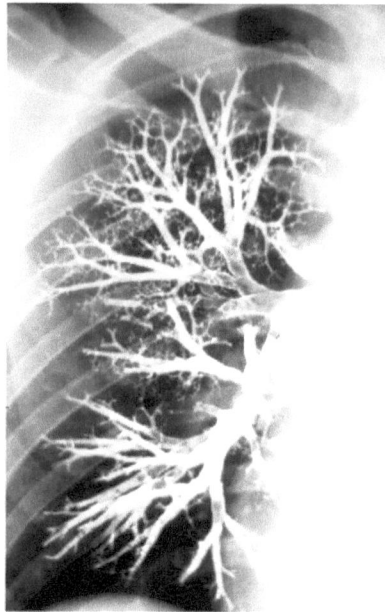

Bronchogram of
tracheal bronchus

References

1. AJR Am J Roentgenol. 1983 Sep;141(3):623. Clinical significance of tracheal bronchus. Harris JH Jr. PMID: 6603784.
2. Benoit Ghaye, MD, David Szapiro, MD, Jean-Marc Fanchamps, MD, and Robert F. Dondelinger, MDRadiographics 2001;21:105-119.
    DOI: http://dx.doi.org/10.1148/radiographics.21.1.g01ja06105.

Question I.24: An emergency surgical tracheotomy is performed in the trauma holding area after unsuccessful attempts at laryngeal intubation.The patient had a respiratory arrest following chemical inhalation injury. Shortly thereafter the nurse declares that the patient's blood pressure is dropping. Chest auscultation reveals decreased breath sound on the right. Oxygen saturation remains stable at 90% on 100% FiO2. The radiology technician is near the room, so a chest radiograph is immediately obtained (shown below). Which of the following is the <u>most likely</u> cause and mechanism of the radiographic finding?

A. Barotrauma from initiation of mechanical ventilation
B. Air entry through the cervical incision
C. Spontaneous rupture of blebs bilaterally

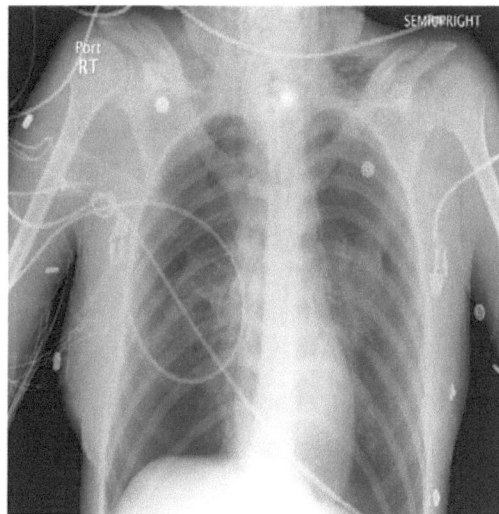

Answer I.24:   B

Synchronous bilateral pneumothorax is a rare but well-documented complication of surgical tracheotomy (1,2). The most likely mechanism for this complication is the entry of air through the cervical incision, and downward passage of air along the outer wall of the trachea into the mediastinum, most likely during inspiration (drop in pleural pressure). One animal study suggested that hyperextension of the neck applies mechanical tension to the mediastinal pleura which might prompt rupture of blebs. Another potential contributory mechanism is marked negative intrapleural pressure during forced inspiration in patients with significant upper airway obstruction (3).

References

1. Tokur M, Kürkçüoðlu IC, Kurul C, Demircan S. Synchronous bilateral pneumothorax as a complication of tracheostomy. Turkish Resp J 2006;7:84-85.
2. Jain S., Deshmukh P, Gaurkar S. Bilateral pneumothorax: Perils of emergency tracheostomy. J Laryngol Voice 2014;4:36-38.
3. Padovan IF, Dawson CA, Henschel EO, Lehman RH. Pathogenesis of mediastinal emphysema and pneumothorax following tracheotomy. Chest 1974;66:553-556.

Question I.25: Which of the following statements best applies to flexible bronchoscopy in an adult patient with severe acute asthma (also known as status asthmaticus)?

A. Multiple studies report a failure of bronchoscopy to help alleviate mucous plugging in critically ill, mechanically ventilated patients with severe acute asthma refractory to medications.
B. In some instances, bronchoscopy with washing may be helpful in improving ventilation in patients with severe acute asthma refractory to medications. Careful monitoring of airway pressures, tidal volume, hemodynamics, and gas exchange is warranted in each instance.
C. Bronchoscopy does not particularly increase the risk of barotrauma and hypoxemia in mechanically ventilated patients with acute severe asthma.

Answer I.25:   B

In some instances bronchoscopy can be helpful in mechanically ventilated patients with acute severe asthma (1-3), but risks and benefits of the procedure must be carefully weighed (4). Bronchoconstriction, mucosal edema, thick, tenacious secretions, mucus plugs, and air trapping increase the risk for barotraumas, hypoxemia, hemodynamic collapse, and death. Precautions include using a bronchoscope with a diameter that is 2mm less in diameter than the inner diameter of the endotracheal tube in order to minimize auto positive end-expiratory pressure (auto-PEEP) and doing bronchoscopy in short bursts where the scope is repeatedly removed from the airway between moments of ventilation and oxygenation. Studies reporting the success of bronchoscopy in patients with status asthmaticus are anecdotal or very small series case reports. There are no specific asthma treatment guidelines that advocate the use of bronchoscopy in patients with severe acute asthma.

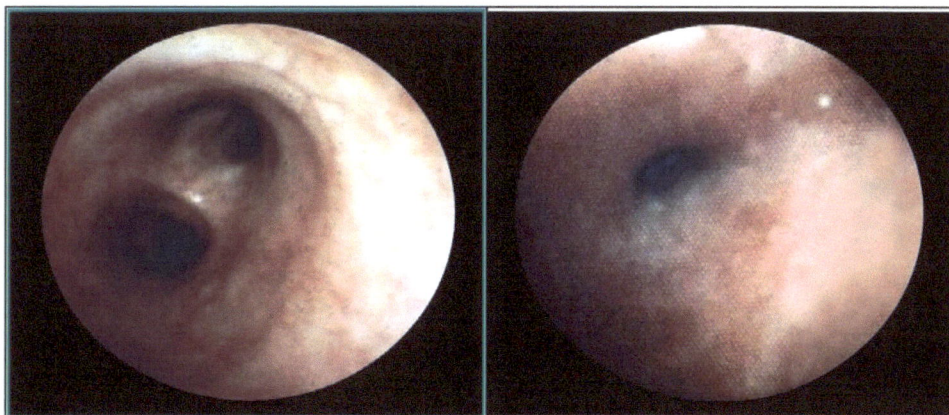

Asthma: Normal airway   Asthma: status asthmaticus

References

1. Maggi JC, Nussbaum E, Babbitt C, Maggi FE, Randhawa I. Pediatric fiberoptic bronchoscopy as adjunctive therapy in acute asthma with respiratory failure. Pediatr Pulmonol. 2012; 47:1180–1184.
2. Durward A, Forte V, Shemie SD. Resolution of mucus plugging and atelectasis after intratracheal rhDNase therapy in a mechanically ventilated child with refractory status asthmaticus. Crit Care Med. 2000; 28:560–562.
3. Khan MF, Al Otair HA, Elgishy AF, Alzeer AH. Bronchoscopy as a rescue therapy in patients with status asthmaticus: Two case reports and review of literature. Saudi J Anaesth. 2013; 7:327–330.
4. Bush A. Primum non nocere: How to cause chaos with a bronchoscope in the ICU. Chest. 2009; 135:2–4.

Question I.26: One day after rigid bronchoscopy and bilateral silicone stent insertion, a critically ill patient with bronchogenic carcinoma and a recent history of left and right main bronchial obstruction complains of increasing dyspnea at rest. What is the <u>most likely</u> cause for his symptoms?

A. Stent obstruction with secretions
B. Pulmonary embolism
C. Stent migration

Answer I.26:   A

   The most likely diagnosis of increasing dyspnea after silicone stent insertion is obstruction by accumulated secretions. This is more likely than granulation tissue formation or migration, especially in patients with indwelling stents in the main bronchi. Inspection bronchoscopy is warranted in stented patients with new or increasing symptoms such as cough or dyspnea. Saline lavage and aspiration will help clear the stents of secretions. Specimens should be sent for microbiology, and antibiotic treatment initiated if infectious organisms are found. Anecdotally, early mobilization and saline nebulization help prevent obstruction. In one study of 23 articles involving 501 patients, authors found stent-associated respiratory tract infection in 20 % of stented patients (1). The most common infection was pneumonia, and most common organisms were *Staphylococcus aureus* and *Pseudomonas aeruginosa* (2).

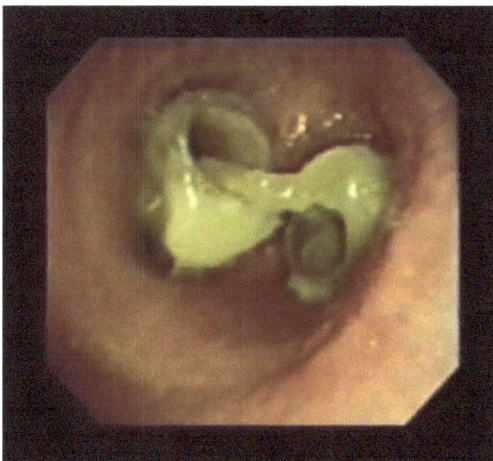

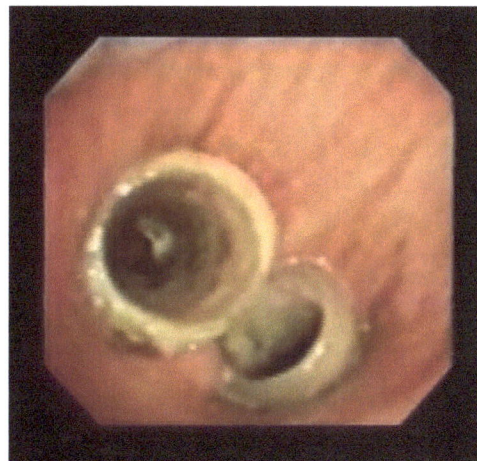

References

1. Agrafiotis M, Siempos I, Falagas ME. Infections related to airway stenting: a systematic review. Respiration. 2009;78(1):69-74.

2. Colt HG, Murgu S. Bronchoscopy in central airway obstruction: A patient-centered approach. Elsevier pub, 2012.

Question 1.27: Four weeks after tracheostomy, a patient has increasing blood and blood-tinged secretions during tracheal suctioning. Flexible bronchoscopy through the tracheostomy tube reveals the image below. What should be the next step?

A. Mobilize the tracheostomy tube in order to see whether the bleeding granulation tissue protruding through the fenestrations of the tracheostomy tube is obstructive in nature.
B. Refer the patient for laser ablation or bronchoscopic electrosurgery to remove the bleeding granulation tissue partially obstructing the fenestration of the tracheostomy tube.
C. Tell the nurses and respiratory therapists to stop tracheal suctioning because the suction catheter causes bleeding each time it strikes the granulation tissue.

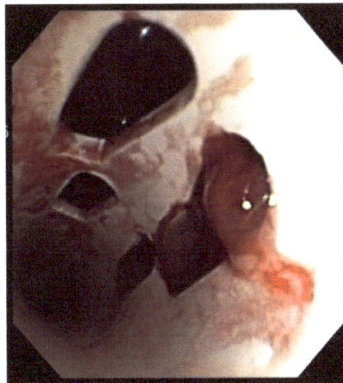

Answer 1.27:   A

Fenestrated tracheostomy tubes are used as a step before complete removal of tracheostomy tubes. It allows a trial of normal breathing and coughing up secretions. It also allows speech by letting air move between the tracheostomy tube and the vocal cords. Granulation tissue can form along the posterior wall of the trachea, growing through the fenestrations into the tracheal tube lumen. This tissue is usually friable and bleeds easily, especially after repeated trauma as caused by frequent suctioning. As the tube is mobilized (manually, but also during deglutition), tissues may move into and out of the fenestration. Moving the tube slightly (under direct bronchoscopic guidance) will allow greater inspection of the size and extent of granulation tissue. Halting the trauma often results in spontaneous resolution. Obstructing or persistently bleeding lesions, however, will require cauterization or removal using bronchoscopic resectional therapies such as laser, electrosurgery, argon plasma, or cryotherapy.

Question I.28: A middle-aged woman with severe chronic obstructive lung disease (emphysema) was hospitalized with severe hypercapnic respiratory failure. Mechanical ventilation is required for 30 days with multiple failed attempts at weaning. There is significant hyperinflation. Comorbidities excluded her from lung transplantation. Which of the following is the most reasonable next step?

A. Inform the family of the dismal prognosis and initiate withdrawal from mechanical ventilation and comfort care.
B. Consult interventional pulmonology to discuss compassionate use of a bronchoscopic lung reduction procedure (valve insertion).
C. Transfer the patient to a long-term ventilator management facility.
D. All of the above

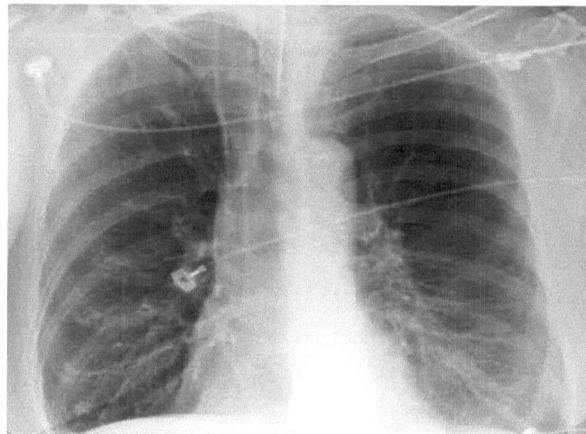

Answer I.28:   D

All of the responses are potentially correct, and of course, management must be individualized based on resources and patient preferences. Endobronchial lung volume reduction is usually reserved for stable patients, but several specialists report anecdotal success using valves on mechanically ventilated patients with severe hyperinflation and low forced expiratory volume. Endobronchial lung volume reduction (ELVR), using one-way valves is a "one-way blocking technique" of ELVR in which the most emphysematous lobe of the lung is occluded by one-way valves (1). Patient selection criteria include heterogeneous emphysema, fissure completeness, and no bronchial thickness. Valves are placed in one or more segmental bronchi in order to close all segments of the involved lobe so that air is allowed to exit during expiration, but not allowed to enter during inspiration. High-resolution computer tomography scans and special software allows precise assessment of the degree of the degree, location, and distribution of hyperventilation and lung destruction (2). Complications from valve insertion include migration (4.7%), hemoptysis (6.1%), and pneumothorax (20 %) (3, 4).

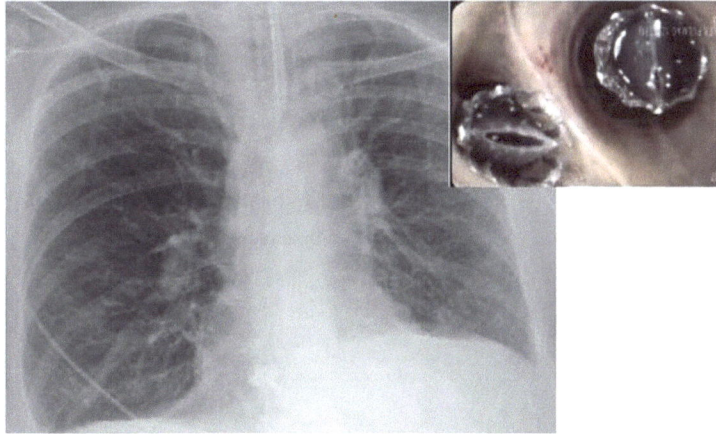

Insertion of bronchial valves in Left upper lobe results in significant volume reduction (note elevation left hemidiaphragm)

References

1. Ralf Eberhardt, Daniela Gompelmann, Felix JF Herth, and Maren Schuhmann. Endoscopic bronchial valve treatment: patient selection and special considerations. Int J Chron Obstruct Pulmon Dis. 2015; 10: 2147–2157.
2. Sciurba FC, Ernst A, Herth FJ, et al. A randomized study of endobronchial valves for advanced emphysema. N Engl J Med.2010;363(13):1233–1244
3. Gompelmann D, Eberhardt R, Herth FJ. Endoscopic lung volume reduction. A European perspective. Ann Am Thorac Soc. 2013;10(6):657–666.
4. Valipour A, Slebos DK, Oliveira H, Eberhardt R, Freitag L, Criner G, Herth F. Expert Statement: Pneumothorax Associated with Endoscopic Valve Therapy for Emphysema - Potential Mechanisms, Treatment Algorithm, and Case Examples. Respiration (English Edition), v. 87, p. 513-521, 2014

Question I.29: A 62-year-old woman with cirrhosis and ruptured right lung abscess develops significant subcutaneous emphysema while on mechanical ventilation. The patient is not a candidate for open surgical repair and conservative measures to stop the air leak have failed repeatedly. A Fogarty balloon is used to isolate the area, which appears to be located in the territory of the right lower lobe lateral-basal (RB9). Which of the following bronchoscopic procedures might be attempted in this patient?

A. Bronchoscopic valve insertion
B. Administration of fibrin glue
C. Watanabe bronchial spigot insertion
D. All of the above

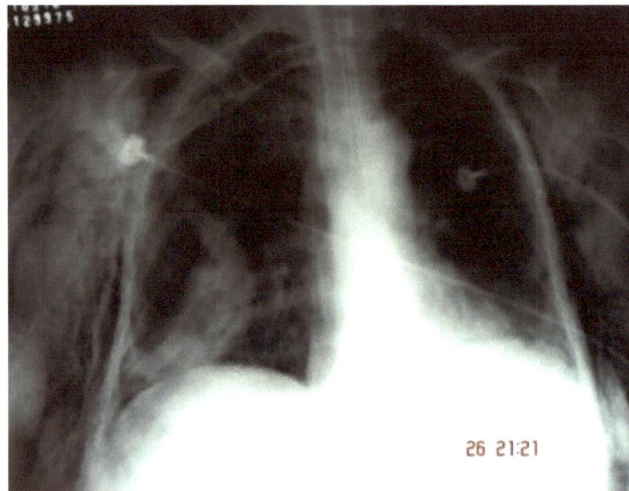

Answer I.29:   D

Many patients with a prolonged air leak and patients with pneumothorax-related difficulties during mechanical ventilation are candidates for bronchoscopic therapy. Although these techniques are not always successful, specialists report relative success in many cases, and several publications report good success of various modalities (understanding, of course, that many cases of negative outcomes might not be reported). Endobronchial valves are usually reserved for patients undergoing bronchoscopic lung volume reduction, but have also been used in cases of pneumothorax, as well as to control bleeding (1-4). Fibrin (cyanoacrylate) glue is a frequently used technique that is occasionally successful (5), but care must be taken to correctly identify the segmental territory and to not damage the bronchoscope at the time of glue administration. The silicone Watanabe spigot has also been used successfully but requires rigid bronchoscopy for insertion (6).

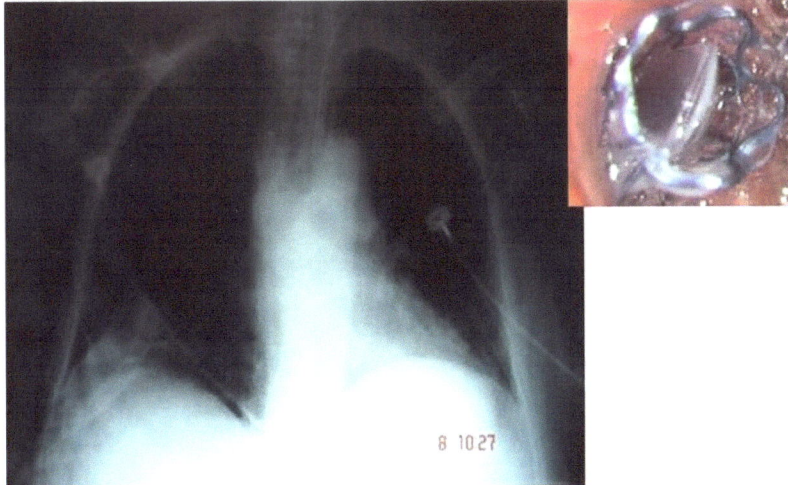

Chest radiograph after insertion of bronchial valve in laterbasal segment of Right lower lobe (RB9) identified after Fogarty balloon isolation (valve seen in closed position)

Watanabe spigot (Novatec)

References

1. Mahajan AK, Verhoef P, Patel SB, et al. A Case Series Describing a Minimally Invasive Approach to Bronchopleural Fistulas in Medical Intensive Care Unit Patients. J Bronchology Interv Pulmonol. 2012 Apr; 19(2): 137–141.
2. Fann JI, Berry GJ, Burdon TA. The use of endobronchial valve device to eliminate air leak. Respiratory Medicine 2006;100 (8):1402–1406.
3. Valle ELT, Oliveira HG, Macedo N, et al. Closure Of Multiple Bronchopleural Fistulas With One-Way Endobronchial Valves: A Minimally Invasive Option For Tuberculosis Complications. American Journal of Respiratory and Critical Care Medicine 2011.A43:1-3.
4. Lalla U1, Allwood BW, Sinha Roy S, et al. Endobronchial Valve Used as Salvage Therapy in a Mechanically Ventilated Patient with Intractable Life-Threatening Hemoptysis. Respiration. 2017 Mar 30. doi: 10.1159/000465526. [Epub ahead of print]

5. Chawla RK, Madan A, Bhardwaj PK, et al Bronchoscopic management of bronchopleural fistula with intrabronchial instillation of glue (N-butyl cyanoacrylate) Lung India. 2012 Jan-Mar; 29(1): 11–14. doi: 10.4103/0970-2113.92350.
6. Watanabe Y, Matsuo K, Tamaoki A, et al. Bronchial Occlusion with Endobronchial Watanabe Spigot. Journal of Bronchology 2003;10(4):264-267.

Question I.30: A patient with known benign tracheal stenosis was treated by insertion of a Montgomery T-tube at another facility. He is transferred to your intensive care unit with a history of recurrent hemoptysis. Flexible bronchoscopy reveals the following image. Which of the following statements is correct about Montgomery T-tubes?

A. Montgomery T-tubes should usually be left closed (using a removable plug) so that patients breathe normally through their trachea and larynx.
B. Montgomery T-tubes are easily connected to Ambu bags in case assisted ventilation is needed.
C. Montgomery T-tubes can only be removed under general anesthesia.

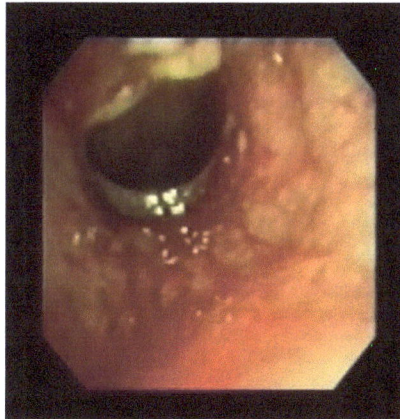

Answer I.30:   A

    The Montgomery T-tube consists of an intratracheal limb with tapered ends to minimize injury to the tracheal mucus membrane (1). The extratracheal limb of the T-tube usually has a plug so that when closed, patients can breathe through their trachea and larynx. This is how T-tubes should usually be used. When fitted appropriately patients can phonate and talk with a T-tube in place. When open, however, the larynx is bypassed and a tracheal airway is assured.

    Montgomery T-tubes are placed in patients with benign tracheal strictures as well as after tracheolaryngeal surgery (2, 3). Because of the proximity of its proximal portion to the undersurface of the vocal cords, granulation tissue formation can be obstructive or bleed easily with phonation, deglutition, or after suction trauma. T-tubes also must be regularly suctioned and kept clean, especially if they are left unplugged for long periods; otherwise, there is risk of obstruction with impacted secretions, which can be life-threatening. A Montgomery T-tube can be removed without anesthesia, especially in an emergency situation, to restore a tracheal airway through the stoma in case of impaction or total obstruction of one of the limbs of the tube. The extratracheal limb of the tube is grasped, and the tube is pulled out using gentle slightly tugging/twisting movements. Ideally, removal should be practiced in models. After emergency removal, it may be necessary to insert a tracheotomy tube, or endotracheal tube via the tracheostomy stoma to maintain and assure airway patency and ventilation.

Montgomery T-tube obstruction may require bronchoscopic resection using electrocautery, argon plasma, cryotherapy, or laser. Risk of airway fires exist if thermal energy technologies are employed (electrocautery, argon plasma, or laser) so necessary precautions regarding resection technique and oxygenation should be used.

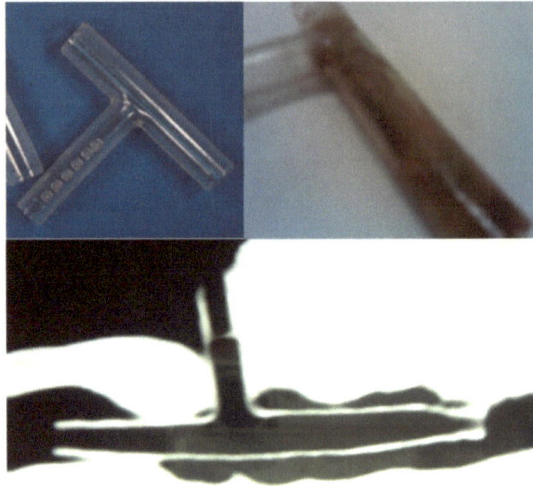

Montgomery T-Tube, Tube obstructed by
secretions, radiograph of tube in airway)

References

1. Montgomery WW. Manual for care of the Montgomery silicone tracheal T-tube. *Ann Otol Rhinol Laryngol* 1980; 89:1-7.
2. Carretta A, Casiraghi M, Melloni G, et al. Montgomery T-tube placement in the treatment of benign tracheal lesions.
3. Eur J Cardiothorac Surg. 2009;36(2):352-356. Guha, S. M. Mostafa, J. B. Kendall. The Montgomery T-tube: anesthetic problems and solutions. Br J Anaesth (2001) 87 (5): 787-790.

***

CONGRATULATIONS

You have now completed Module I of The Essential Intensivist Bronchoscopist©.

The following section contains a ten question post-test and answers.

Post-tests are True/False. Please remember that while many programs consider 70% correct responses a passing grade, the student's "target" score should be 100%.

Please send us your opinion regarding Bronchoscopy Education Project materials by contacting your national bronchology association or emailing us at www.bronchoscopy.org.

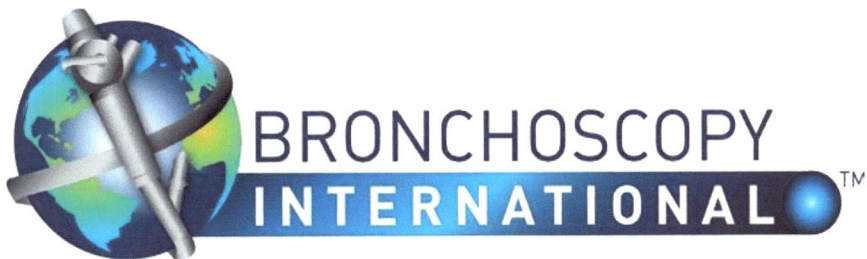

MODULE I

TEN QUESTION TRUE/FALSE POST-TEST

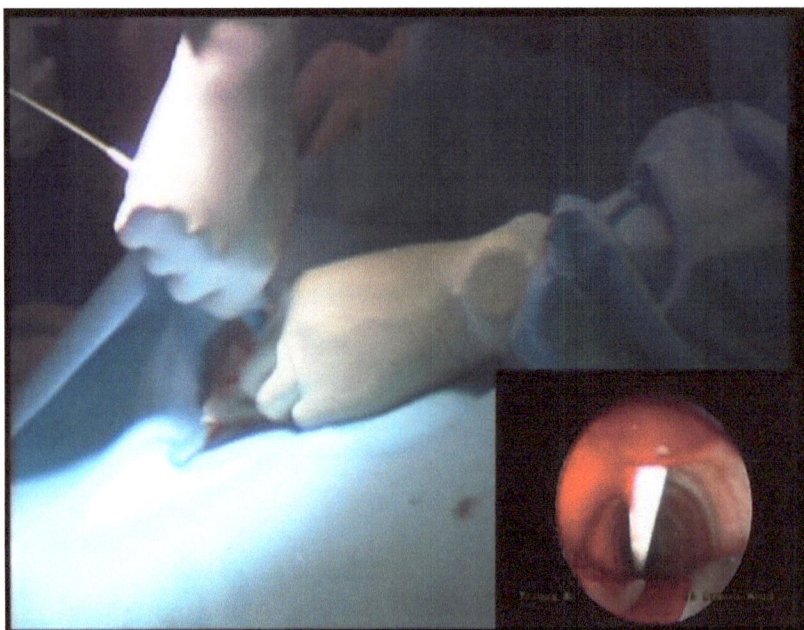

The Essential Intensivist Bronchoscopist

Module I Post-test

INSTRUCTIONS: Answer True or False to each of the following <u>TEN</u> questions.

Question 1: Work of breathing improves and peak inspiratory pressures decrease in patients with tracheostomy tubes as compared with endotracheal tubes.

Question 2: The 4th-5th intercartilaginous space is an ideal site for percutaneous tracheostomy tube placement.

Question 3: At least one randomized control trial shows that single-step dilatational technique is superior to other techniques for percutaneous tracheostomy.

Question 4: Tracheal strictures (identified as more than 10 percent narrowing of the airway lumen) are expected in about thirty percent of patients after percutaneous tracheostomy.

Question 5: Wound infection appears to occur less frequently after percutaneous tracheostomy than after open surgical tracheostomy.

Question 6: Impacted secretions, infection, migration, and granulation tissue formation are known complications of both silicone and metal airway stents.

Question 7: Bronchoscopy is rarely needed to diagnose airway complications in mechanically ventilated patients or in those with a tracheotomy.

Question 8: Montgomery T-tubes require surveillance because of the risk of subglottic granulation tissue formation, and impacted secretions if the stoma limb is left open.

Question 9: In addition to migration risks, endobronchial valves may cause pneumothorax and hemoptysis in bronchoscopic lung volume reduction patients.

Question 10: Morbid obesity is a well-known contraindication to percutaneous tracheostomy.

***

Answers to

The Essential Intensivist Bronchoscopist

post-test Module I

ANSWERS

1: True
2: False
3: True
4: True
5: True
6: True
7: False
8: True
9: True
10: False

TOTAL SCORE _____/10

MODULE II

THIRTY MULTIPLE CHOICE QUESTION/ANSWER SETS

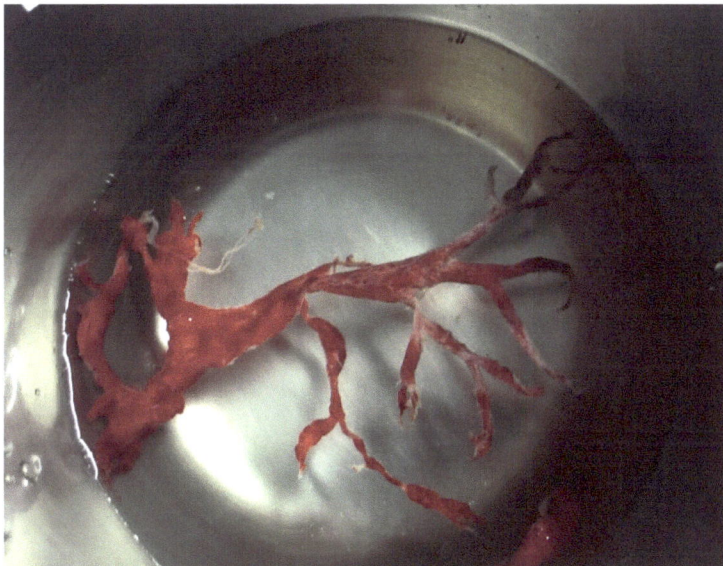

The Essential Intensivist Bronchoscopist©

The Essential Intensivist Bronchoscopist MODULE II

LEARNING OBJECTIVES

After completing this module the reader should be able to:

1. Describe at least three therapeutic applications of flexible bronchoscopy in cases of respiratory failure due to central airway obstruction.
2. Describe the indications and contraindications for performing bronchoscopy using non-invasive mechanical positive pressure ventilation (NIPPV).
3. Identify and describe the role of bronchoscopy in cases of atelectasis, aspiration pneumonia, ventilator-associated pneumonia, and acute respiratory distress imitators.
4. Describe at least three techniques for managing massive hemoptysis in the intensive care unit.
5. List at least five potential complications of bronchoscopy in critically ill patients (including those with elevated intracranial pressure, severe hypoxemia, hypercarbia, asthma, tracheal stenosis, and advanced emphysema).

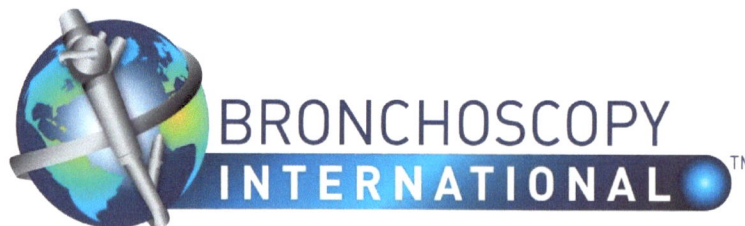

Question II.1: Patients with increased intracranial pressure (ICP) herniated during flexible fiberoptic bronchoscopy (FFB). This statement is:

A.   True
B.   False

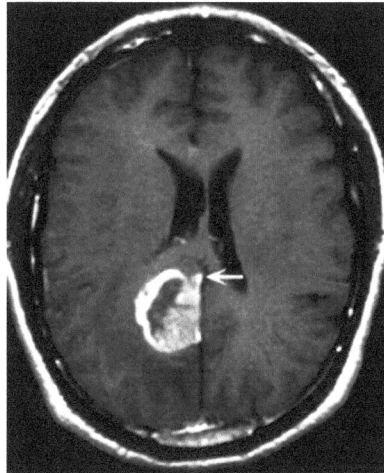

Answer II.1:   B

It is usually safe to perform bronchoscopy in these patients. The increased intracranial pressure (ICP) during bronchoscopy is matched by an increase in mean arterial pressure (MAP) which maintains cerebral perfusion pressure (CPP).

A prospective study was done to assess the effect of bronchoscopy on ICP and CPP in patients with brain injuries (1). After the introduction of the scope, the mean ICP which was 12.6 mm Hg at baseline rapidly increased in 81% of the patients, to the highest ICP of 38.0 mm Hg. There was, however, a concomitant increase in the MAP such that there was no substantial change in CPP. The average time for the return of ICP to baseline was 13.9 minutes. No patient had acute neurologic deterioration secondary to bronchoscopy as evidenced by the fact that no patient demonstrated persistent intracranial hypertension or developed acute herniation. Bajwa et al evaluated this risk by reviewing hospital records of twenty-nine patients who had CT evidence of increased ICP (2). Patients were divided into two groups: group 1 with 17 patients had evidence of raised ICP prior to the performance of bronchoscopy and had received 6 days of pretreatment with an intent to lower the ICP, and group 2 with 12 patients in whom increased ICP was not suspected at the time of bronchoscopy and therefore did not receive any form of pretreatment. There was no evidence of neurologic complications in either group during the first week after bronchoscopy.

In another study, the effect of bronchoscopy on cerebral hemodynamics in patients with severe head injury was determined (3). During bronchoscopy, patients experienced a mean increase in ICP of 13.5 mm Hg above basal values. At peak ICP, MAP increased from a baseline of 92.3 mm Hg (SD +/- 16.1) to 111.5 mm Hg (+/- 13.9). Mean CPP was 83.7 mm Hg at peak ICP (range, 52 to 121 mm Hg), a 14.0% increase over baseline. The ICP and MAP returned to basal levels following bronchoscopy. No patient had a clinically significant increase in ICP or demonstrated any deterioration in Glasgow Coma Scale score or neurologic examination findings post-bronchoscopy.

Although bronchoscopy causes an increase in ICP in patients with severe head injury, the MAP also rises, and an adequate CPP is usually maintained. The ICP returns to basal levels after the procedure. When properly performed, bronchoscopy does not adversely affect neurologic status in patients with severe head injury.

References

1. Kerwin AJ, Croce MA, Timmons SD, Maxwell RA, Malhotra AK, Fabian TC. Effects of fiberoptic bronchoscopy on intracranial pressure in patients with brain injury: a prospective clinical study. J Trauma 2000; 48(5): 878-82; discussion 882-3.
2. Bajwa MK, Henein S, Kamholz SL. Fiberoptic bronchoscopy in the presence of space-occupying intracranial lesions. Chest 1993; 104(1): 101-3.
3. Peerless JR, Snow N, Likavec MJ, Pinchak AC, Malangoni MA. The effect of fiberoptic bronchoscopy on cerebral hemodynamics in patients with severe head injury. Chest 1995; 108(4): 962-5.

Question II.2: Severe hypoxemia is a contraindication to flexible bronchoscopy (FB) in the non-intubated patient. This statement is:

A. True
B. False

Answer II.2: B

Severe hypoxemia is not a contraindication to bronchoscopy in the non-intubated patient, but precautions are necessary. Noninvasive positive pressure ventilation (NPPV) may improve oxygenation, thus allowing bronchoscopy in the severely hypoxemic non-intubated patient. Antonelli et al. evaluated the feasibility and safety of NPPV via a face mask during FB with bronchoalveolar lavage (BAL) in immunosuppressed patients with gas exchange abnormalities that would otherwise contraindicate using conventional unassisted FB (1). Inclusion criteria included the following: PaO_2/fraction of inspired oxygen (FIO_2) of 100 or less; pH of 7.35 or more; and improvement in oxygen (O_2) saturation during NPPV before initiating FB. A full-face mask was connected to a ventilator (Servo 900C; Solna, Sweden) set to deliver continuous positive airway pressure (CPAP) of 4 cm H_2O, pressure support ventilation of 17 cm H_2O, and 1.0 FIO_2. The mask was secured to the patient with head straps. NPPV began 10 min before starting FB and continued for 90 min or more after the procedure was completed. NPPV significantly improved PaO_2/FIO_2 and O_2 saturation. FB with NPPV was well tolerated, and no patient required endotracheal intubation. In another study, also performed by Antonelli et al, the efficacy of using NPPV to assist spontaneous breathing in patients with less severe forms of hypoxemia (i.e., PaO_2/FIO_2 ratio < 200) was evaluated by comparing it with conventional oxygen supplementation via Venturi mask (2). During FB, the mean PaO_2/FIO_2 ratio increased by 82% in the NPPV and decreased by 10% in the conventional oxygen supplementation group. Sixty minutes after undergoing FB, the NPPV group had a higher mean PaO_2/FIO_2 ratio, a lower mean heart rate and no reduction in mean arterial pressure in comparison to a 15% decrease from the baseline in the control group. One patient in the NPPV group and two patients in the control group required non-emergent intubation. Authors considered that intubation was due to disease worsening. The tolerance of FB without and with CPAP, delivered through a full-face mask was compared in severe hypoxemic ($PaO_2 < 125$ mm Hg under a high FIO_2 mask driven by 10 L/min oxygen) (3). Thirty patients were enrolled in the study, with 15 patients in each group. During the 6 h after FB, eight patients required mechanical ventilation ventilatory support: seven in the oxygen group and one patient in the CPAP group. Five patients in the oxygen group, but none in the CPAP group, developed respiratory failure attributed to FB in the 6 h after FB and required mechanical ventilation.

In conclusion, as long as oxygenation can be improved to > 92% oxygen saturation, hypoxemia alone is not a contraindication to diagnostic FB. NPPV improves lung mechanics, oxygenation and might prevent intubation in these high-risk patients.

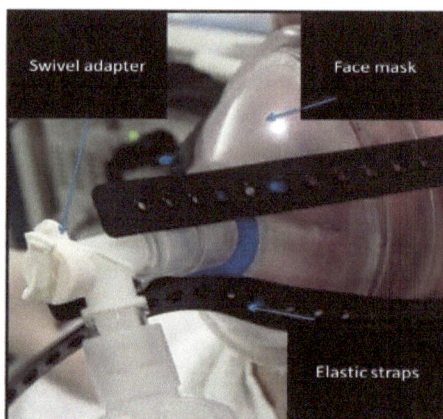

References

1. Antonelli M, Conti G, Riccioni L, Meduri GU. Noninvasive positive-pressure ventilation via face mask during bronchoscopy with BAL in high-risk hypoxemic patients. Chest 1996; 110(3): 724-8.
2. Antonelli M, Conti G, Rocco M, Arcangeli A, Cavaliere F, Proietti R, Meduri GU. Noninvasive positive-pressure ventilation vs. conventional oxygen supplementation in hypoxemic patients undergoing diagnostic bronchoscopy. Chest 2002; 121(4): 1149-54.
3. Maitre B, Jaber S, Maggiore SM, Bergot E, Richard JC, Bakthiari H, Housset B, Boussignac G, Brochard L. Continuous positive airway pressure during fiberoptic bronchoscopy in hypoxemic patients. A randomized double-blind study using a new device. Am J Respir Crit Care Med 2000; 162(3 Pt 1): 1063-7.

Question II.3: A patient with severe emphysema has developed mucus plugging with complete right lung atelectasis due to community-acquired pneumonia (CAP). He has a history of congestive heart failure, chronic CO_2 retention and now he's awake, in mild distress, follows commands and using 100% non re-breather mask with an O_2 sat of 97%. Chest physical therapy, suctioning, bronchodilators and mucolytics failed to improve the chest radiograph. A bronchoscopy for therapeutic aspiration is being considered. What should be done next?

A.   Intubate for the procedure
B.   Place patient on BIPAP and proceed with bronchoscopy
C.   Continue conservative management

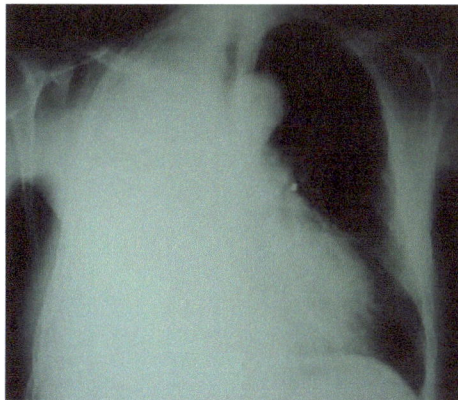

Answer II.3:   B

Noninvasive positive pressure ventilation (NPPV) assistance is a satisfactory alternative to endotracheal intubation in many patients with severe refractory hypoxemia, severe COPD, postoperative respiratory failure, or severe obstructive sleep apnea and obesity hypoventilation syndrome who require flexible bronchoscopy for diagnostic or therapeutic purposes (1). NPPV improves gas exchange and work of breathing by reducing intrapulmonary shunt and ventilation-perfusion mismatch. These effects are primarily a result of recruitment of collapsed alveoli by positive end-expiratory pressure.

One study assessed the feasibility and safety of NPPV via a face mask during flexible bronchoscopy (FB) in patients with severe COPD, often considered a relative contraindication to FB during spontaneous ventilation (2). Inclusion criteria were: PaO_2 <70 mmHg despite nasal O_2 delivered at 3 Lt/min, $PaCO_2$> 50 mmHg, and improvement of SpO_2 with NPPV before FB. Patients had no signs of acute respiratory failure, were admitted to the intensive care unit for pneumonia, and required a bronchoalveolar lavage (BAL). No patient required endotracheal intubation within 24 hours and there was no mortality. Application of NPPV during FB is considered a safe technique for maintaining adequate gas exchange in hypoxemic and hypercapnic COPD patients who are not in acute respiratory failure. After the end of the procedure, close monitoring in the intensive care unit is essential.

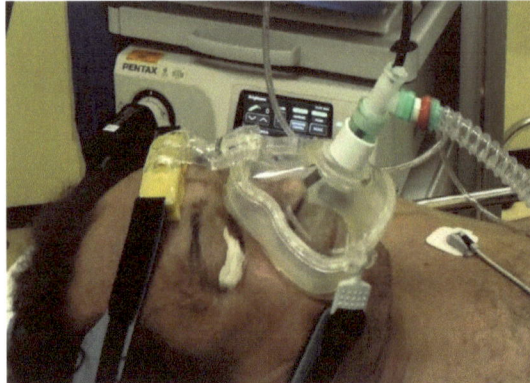

References

1. Murgu SD, Pecson J, Colt HG. Flexible bronchoscopy assisted by noninvasive positive pressure ventilation. Crit Care Nurse 2011; 31(3): 70-6.
2. Da Conceiçao M, Genco G, Favier JC, Bidallier I, Pitti R. [Fiberoptic bronchoscopy during noninvasive positive-pressure ventilation in patients with chronic obstructive lung disease with hypoxemia and hypercapnia]. Ann Fr Anesth Reanim 2000; 19(4): 231-6.

Question II.4: A patient with a remote history of stroke had an acute aspiration event. The patient developed hypoxemic respiratory failure and was placed on mechanic ventilation (MV); FiO_2 80%; PEEP 12 cm H_2O. The medical ICU team calls you to perform a bronchoscopy as soon as possible. You should:

A.   Do it!
B.   Don't do it!

Answer II.4:   A

A retrospective cohort study evaluated the therapeutic role of early bronchoscopy in patients with aspiration pneumonia who were mechanically ventilated (1). Patients who underwent bronchoscopy within 24 hours after intubation were categorized as the early bronchoscopy group (n=93) and the others as the late bronchoscopy group. Of the 154 patients who were included in the study, the early bronchoscopy group showed significantly lower intensive care unit (ICU) and 90-day mortality (ICU: 4.9% vs. 24.6%; 90-day: 11.8 vs 32.8%) regardless of the initial empirical antibiotics. In addition, their sequential organ failure assessment score on day 7 tended to decrease more rapidly. Among the survivors, patients in the early bronchoscopy group were extubated earlier, with a higher success rate, had a shorter length of mechanical ventilation and had a shorter ICU stay. It was concluded that early bronchoscopy could benefit the clinical outcomes of mechanically ventilated patients with aspiration pneumonia.

References

1. Lee HW, Min J, Park J, Lee YJ, Kim SJ, Park JS, Yoon HI, Lee JH, Lee CT, Cho YJ. Clinical impact of early bronchoscopy in mechanically ventilated patients with aspiration pneumonia. Respirology 2015; 20(7): 1115-22.

Question II.5: Bronchoscopic interventions for diagnosing ventilator-associated pneumonia (VAP) in immunocompetent patients improve outcomes. This statement is:

A.   True
B.   False

Answer II.5:   B

VAP is common in intensive care units (ICUs). The efficacy of quantitative cultures of respiratory secretions and invasive strategies in reducing mortality in immunocompetent patients with VAP, compared with qualitative cultures and non-invasive strategies was evaluated in one systematic review (1). Five randomized controlled trials (RCTs) (1367 patients) compared respiratory samples processed quantitatively or qualitatively, obtained by invasive or non-invasive methods from immunocompetent patients with VAP; authors analyzed the impact of these methods on antibiotic use and mortality rates. The studies that compared quantitative and qualitative cultures (1240 patients) showed no statistically significant differences in mortality rates.

The analysis of all five RCTs showed there was no evidence of a reduction in mortality in the invasive group versus the non-invasive group. There were no significant differences between the interventions with respect to the number of days on mechanical ventilation, length of ICU stay or antibiotic change. There was no evidence that the use of quantitative cultures of respiratory secretions results in reduced mortality, reduced time in ICU and on mechanical ventilation, or higher rates of antibiotic change when compared to qualitative cultures in patients with VAP. Similar results were observed when invasive strategies were compared with non-invasive strategies. Thus, bronchoscopy with bronchoalveolar lavage (BAL) cannot be routinely recommended to diagnose VAP.

References

1. Berton DC, Kalil AC, Teixeira PJ. Quantitative versus qualitative cultures of respiratory secretions for clinical outcomes in patients with ventilator-associated pneumonia. Cochrane Database Syst Rev 2014; 10: CD006482.

Question II.6: A patient with ventilator-associated pneumonia (VAP) (*Pseudomonas Aeruginosa* on cultures) developed new left lower lobe atelectasis on day 7 since initiation of mechanic ventilation (MV). Oxygenation requirement increased, PEEP was increased from 8 to 12 and FiO_2 was increased from 0.4 to 0.6. You are called to perform a bronchoscopy for therapeutic aspiration of secretions. You should:

A.   Do it!

B.   Don't do it!

Answer II.6:   B

Even though one of the most common indications for bronchoscopy is the presence of retained secretions and atelectasis, there is little research dedicated to its safety and utility in this clinical situation. Atelectasis is a frequent complication seen in the ICU, which may worsen hypoxemia and may predispose the patient to superimposed nosocomial pneumonia. Traditionally, the treatment of atelectasis in ICU patients has focused on suctioning with adjuvant therapy such as chest physiotherapy and bronchoscopy.

Across numerous case series, bronchoscopy has been shown to be moderately effective in removing retained secretions and improving atelectasis, with a wide range of success rates (19 to 89%) depending on the characteristics of the subgroups analyzed (1). Oxygen insufflation may be of additional benefit to bronchoscopy. Case series of insufflation added to bronchoscopy have reported improvement in atelectasis in 70-80% with pressures 30-40 cm H_2O via a three-way stopcock.

To evaluate the usefulness of bronchoscopy for treatment of acute lobar atelectasis, in one study 31 subjects were randomly allocated to bronchoscopy followed by respiratory therapy every 4 hours for 48 hrs (n=14), or to respiratory therapy alone (n=17) every 4 hours, followed by bronchoscopy at 24 hrs if atelectasis has not improved (2). No significant differences were detected in the rate of atelectasis resolution with bronchoscopy vs. chest therapy at either 24 or 48 h. The improvement noted immediately after bronchoscopy was the same as that seen with the initial chest percussion therapy. For both groups, approximately 80% of volume loss noted on the CXR was restored by 24 h. These results suggest that bronchoscopy did not add value to respiratory therapy in the initial treatment of acute lobar atelectasis. İf chest therapy fails, however, and the patient continues to have hypoxemia, therapeutic bronchoscopy for removal of secretions should be considered.

References

1. Kreider ME, Lipson DA. Bronchoscopy for atelectasis in the ICU: a case report and review of the literature. Chest 2003; 124(1): 344-50.

2. Marini JJ, Pierson DJ, Hudson LD. Acute lobar atelectasis: a prospective comparison of fiberoptic bronchoscopy and respiratory therapy. Am Rev Respir Dis 1979; 119(6): 971-8.

Question II.7: 66-year-old man with a history of right pneumonectomy for non-small cell carcinoma (NSCLC), presents with acute respiratory failure requiring intubation due to new distal left main bronchial obstruction. What should be done next?

A.   Laser-assisted tumor debulking
B.   Airway stent insertion
C.   External beam radiation
D.   Comfort care

Answer II.7:   A

The efficacy of emergent rigid bronchoscopic intervention, including Nd: YAG laser resection or stent insertion, and the need for continued mechanical ventilation or intensive care level of support in critically ill patients with acute respiratory failure from malignant or benign central airways obstruction was evaluated in one study (1). Emergent laser resection or stent insertion can favorably affect health-care utilization in patients with acute respiratory distress from central airways obstruction. Treatment may be lifesaving and allows successful removal from mechanical ventilation, hospitalization in a lower level of care environment, relief of symptoms, and extended survival of these critically ill patients.

In patients with regionally advanced cancer, this procedure provides palliation and improves performance status to allow initiation of systemic therapy. Overall, inoperable malignant airway obstruction (MAO) has a poor prognosis but lung function and quality of life can be improved using endobronchial treatment modalities.

References

1. Colt HG, Harrell JH. Therapeutic rigid bronchoscopy allows level of care changes in patients with acute respiratory failure from central airways obstruction. Chest 1997; 112(1): 202-6.

Question II.8: A 59-year-old Asian woman with a remote history of tuberculosis presents with wheezing and dyspnea refractory to asthma treatment and oral corticosteroids. She has stridor and is admitted to medical ICU. Flexible bronchoscopy reveals the images below. The most likely diagnosis is tracheal stenosis complicated by:

A.   Tuberculosis tracheitis
B.   Aspergillus tracheitis

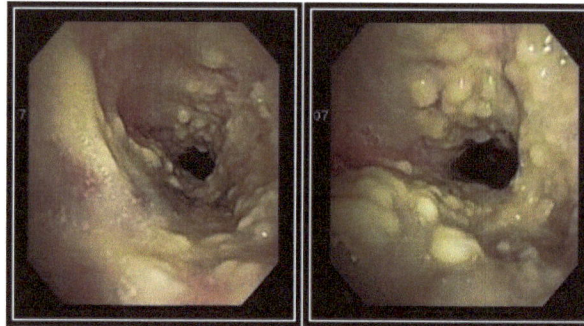

Answer II.8:   B

In reality, either of these two diseases might cause the abnormalities noted in the Figure above, but this was a case of severe Aspergillus infection in a patient with known history of tuberculosis. Aspergillus tracheitis is responsible for less than 7% of all pulmonary aspergillosis. It may be obstructive, ulcerative and pseudomembranous as represented in the Figure below (1). Bronchoscopically, there is usually extensive inflammation with formation of pseudomembranes overlying mucosa containing aspergillus species. Branching, septate fungae are seen on biopsies and washings. Systemic, inhaled antifungals and bronchoscopic management are used for the treatment. Patients are usually treated with antifungal agents such as amphotericin B (conventional, nebulized), liposomal amphotericin or voriconazole. Itraconazole has also been used in non-immunocompromised hosts and as an adjunctive treatment. Bronchoscopic debridement may be warranted in some patients with obstruction from aspergillus pseudomembranous tracheobronchitis.

Aspergillus tracheobronchitis (ATB) is considered as an unusual form of invasive aspergillosis and has a poor outcome. In a prospective study of invasive bronchial-pulmonary aspergillosis (IBPA) in a critically ill COPD population, among 153 critically ill COPD patients admitted to the ICU, eight cases were complicated by ATB [23.5% of invasive bronchial-pulmonary aspergillosis (8 of 34); and 5.2% of COPD (8 of 153)] (2). The overall mortality rate was 72.7%; 77.8% received systemic corticosteroid therapy and 33.3% inhaled corticosteroids before diagnosis with ATB.

Tuberculosis tracheitis can also present in a similar pattern. Forms of endobronchial tuberculosis (EBTB) are classified into seven subtypes by bronchoscopic finding: actively caseating, edematous-hyperemic, fibrostenotic, tumorous, granular, ulcerative, and nonspecific bronchitic. The actively caseating type (43.0%) is the most common form (3). EBTB is highly contagious and seen in ~ 6% of pulmonary TB; 50% of sputum samples are AFB positive and 65% of patients with actively caseating tuberculosis might develop fibrostenosis within 3 months of treatment.

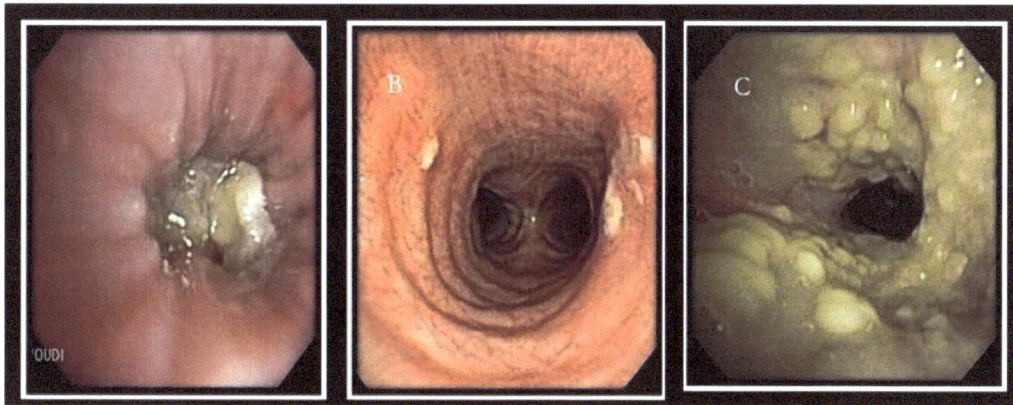

(A) Obstructive   (B) Ulcerative   (C) Pseudomembranous

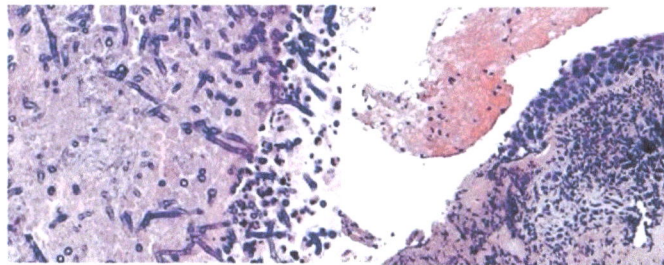

Bronchial washing and biopsies: branching
septate fungal hyphae and necrosis

References

1. Karnak D, Avery RK, Gildea TR, Sahoo D, Mehta AC. Endobronchial fungal disease: an under-recognized entity. Respiration 2007; 74(1): 88-104.
2. He H, Jiang S, Zhang L, Sun B, Li F, Zhan Q, Wang C. Aspergillus tracheobronchitis in critically ill patients with chronic obstructive pulmonary diseases. Mycoses 2014; 57(8): 473-82.
3. Chung HS, Lee JH. Bronchoscopic assessment of the evolution of endobronchial tuberculosis. Chest 2000; 117(2): 385-92.

Question II.9: A 43-year-old woman with asthma refractory to medications develops acute respiratory failure. Bronchoscopy reveals a circumferentially collapsing airway. The Figure below is from the subglottic area. What is the diagnosis?

A.   Relapsing polychondritis
B.   Granulomatosis with polyangiitis
C.   Tracheal amyloidosis
D.   Sarcoidosis

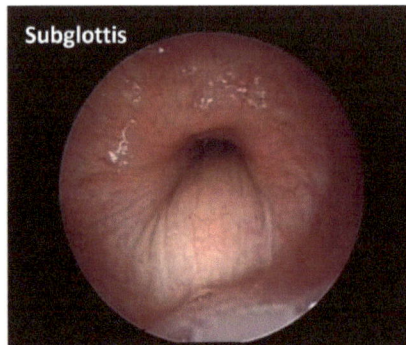

Answer II.9:   A

Relapsing polychondritis is an uncommon, multisystem disease that can be life-threatening and difficult to diagnose (1). On average, it takes three years for diagnosis since first symptoms appear. The illness is of unknown etiology and is characterized by recurrent, potentially severe episodes of inflammation of cartilaginous tissues. All types of cartilage may be involved. Because no specific tests are available, relapsing polychondritis is diagnosed on clinical grounds. Empirical diagnostic criteria proposed by McAdam et al., require three or more clinical features, even without biopsy confirmation (2, 3). These include recurrent chondritis of both auricles, non-erosive inflammatory polyarthritis, chondritis of nose cartilage, inflammation of ocular structures, keratitis, sclerites or uveitis, chondritis of the respiratory tract, laryngeal or tracheal cartilage involvement, and cochlear or vestibular damage causing sensor neural hearing loss, tinnitus or vertigo.

Bronchoscopy is often informative but carries a risk for exacerbating airway inflammation. Intubation for any reason may be difficult because of a small glottis and subglottis caused by edema or cartilage destruction (malacia). In patients without laryngeal involvement, trauma at the time of endotracheal tube insertion may incite localized disease. Because it leads to inflammation of one or more costosternal cartilages, costochondritis may further impair breathing. Involvement of the cartilaginous structures of the respiratory tract is one of the most serious complications of relapsing polychondritis and accounts for 10% to 50% of deaths attributed to this disease. Once malacia develops, steroids don't change the outcome

(2); 50% of deaths are because of respiratory failure. The cellular and humoral response against collagen type II, IX and XI (30-70% of pts) are responsible for the pathogenesis. There can be a delay in diagnosis of approximately 3 years because it is an asthma imitator; more than 50 % of patients have airway involvement and 14% of the patients have respiratory symptoms as the initial presentation; 26% of the patients have subglottic stenosis and 48% of the patients develop Tracheobronchomalacia (TBM). The 5-year survival rate is as low as 45%. Stent insertion, tracheostomy, and CPAP are used for the treatment of TBM related to this disease.

References

1. Trentham DE, Le CH. Relapsing polychondritis. Ann Intern Med 1998129(2)114-22.
2. McAdam LP, O'Hanlan MA, Bluestone R, Pearson CM. Relapsing polychondritis: prospective study of 23 patients and a review of the literature. Medicine (Baltimore) 197655(3): 193-215.
3. Drosos AA. Relapsing polychondritis. Orphanet, 2004: https:// www.orpha.net/data/ patho/GB/uk-RP.pdf

Question II.10: Which of the following is currently considered the most common cause of massive hemoptysis?

A.   Tuberculosis
B.   Lung cancer
C.   Mycetoma
D.   Bronchiectasis

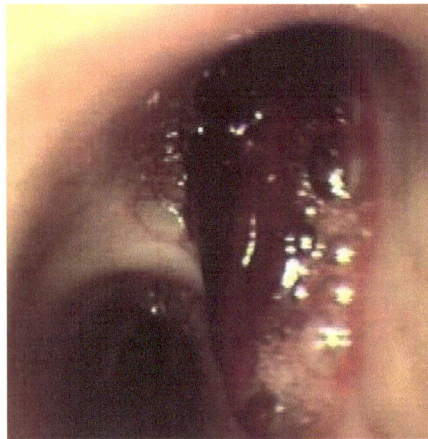

Answer II.10:   D

Currently, bronchiectasis, tuberculosis, mycetomas, necrotizing pneumonia and bronchogenic carcinomas are the main causes of massive hemoptysis (1). In most recent studies, bronchiectasis accounted for the majority of cases of massive hemoptysis. Although hemoptysis is a frequently encountered symptom, massive hemoptysis is always regarded as a potentially lethal condition (1).

Massive hemoptysis may require transfusion and endotracheal intubation; however, blood clots can cause airway obstruction, hypoxemia, and death. Morbidity related to airway bleeding is explained based on physiologic consequences of airway bleeding: blood filling of dead-space (anatomic dead space= 150 ml), airway obstruction and clot formation, subsequent tachypnea and hypoxemia, tachycardia, bradycardia, hypotension, respiratory failure, arrhythmia and cardiac arrest. Underlying disease state (e.g. history of pneumonectomy, critically illness and significant comorbidities) is also very important as respiratory failure may develop even without a large amount of bleeding. Mortality rates from massive hemoptysis have ranged from 9 to 38%.

Bronchovascular fistula is a rare disease mostly seen in the patients with lung transplant-related airway anastomotic ischemic or infectious necrosis, Rasmussen's aneurysms, transbronchial lung biopsy, endobronchial brachytherapy/photodynamic therapy, radiofrequency ablation or cancer. Poor prognosticators of massive hemoptysis are bleeding rate of at least 1,000 ml within a 24-hour, aspiration of blood in the contralateral lung, massive bleeding requiring single-lung ventilation, lung cancer and recurrent bleeding following bronchial artery embolization (BAE).

References

1. Sakr L, Dutau H. Massive hemoptysis: an update on the role of bronchoscopy in diagnosis and management. Respiration 2010; 80(1): 38-58.

Question II.11: Which of the following diagnostic modalities has the highest sensitivity for identifying the cause of massive hemoptysis?

A. Chest radiograph
B. Flexible Bronchoscopy
C. Chest computed tomography

Answer II.11:   C

The aim of the diagnostic strategies for massive hemoptysis is to reveal the underlying cause and localization of the bleeding site. Chest radiography reveals the cause in 35% of cases. Chest computerized tomography (CT) reveals the cause in 60-77% of cases; its sensitivity is 70–88.5% for localization. Bronchoscopy reveals the site of bleeding in 73-93% but sensitivity for identifying the cause is only 2.5-8 %. Radiographic studies (chest radiography and CT) are highly informative to guide the approach to bronchial artery embolization (BAE) and may obviate the need for bronchoscopy in patients with hemoptysis of known etiology, not requiring urgent airway management (1).

References

1. Hsiao EI, Kirsch CM, Kagawa FT, Wehner JH, Jensen WA, Baxter RB. Utility of fiberoptic bronchoscopy before bronchial artery embolization for massive hemoptysis. AJR Am J Roentgenol 2001; 177(4): 861-7.

Question II.12: A patient with a history of tuberculosis presents with massive hemoptysis presumably from a large right upper lobe cavity (seen on a non-contrast chest CT). The patient is admitted to the ICU, where selective intubation of the left main bronchus is performed. Oxygenation is maintained at SpO_2 92-94% of FiO_2 of 0.7. There is no hemodynamic instability. Which of the following is warranted before sending the patient to interventional radiology for bronchial artery embolization (BAE)?

A.   Proceed with bronchial artery embolization
B.   Perform emergent flexible bronchoscopy
C.   Perform a multi-detector chest angiography

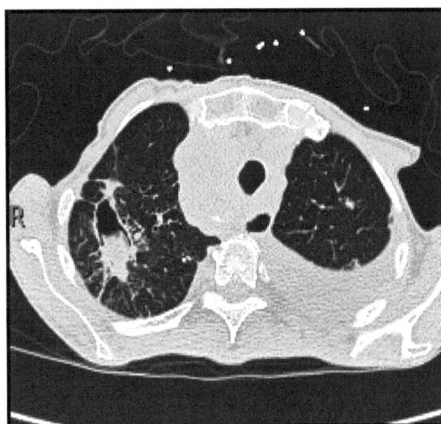

Answer II.12:   **C**

Multidetector-row CT angiography (MDCTA) is an accurate method for distinguishing bronchial from pulmonary artery origin. Signs of pulmonary arterial hemoptysis seen on MDCTA include pseudoaneurysm of the pulmonary artery, aneurysm of the pulmonary artery and the presence of a pulmonary artery in the inner wall of a cavity. MDCTA findings of associated bronchial arterial hypertrophy predict the need for simultaneous bronchial artery and pulmonary artery embolization (1).

Bronchoscopy is useful in cases of bilateral lung opacities (to localize the source) and for endobronchial management in emergent situations. The likelihood of visualizing the site of bleeding is significantly better with early versus delayed bronchoscopy, but it appears that the timing of the procedure does not alter therapeutic decisions or clinical outcome in non-massive hemoptysis (2).

In this patient with nonmassive hemoptysis, stable oxygenation and hemodynamics, and a chest CT that identifies a likely source, a bronchoscopy will probably not add valuable information. Knowing if the source is from a bronchial or pulmonary arterial source, however, affects treatment decisions, and thus a contrast-enhanced chest CT should be performed.

References

1. Khalil A, Parrot A, Nedelcu C, Fartoukh M, Marsault C, Carette MF. Severe hemoptysis of pulmonary arterial origin: signs and role of multidetector row CT angiography. Chest 2008; 133(1): 212-9.
2. Gong H Jr, Salvatierra C. Clinical efficacy of early and delayed fiberoptic bronchoscopy in patients with hemoptysis. Am Rev Respir Dis 1981; 124(3): 221-5.

Question II.13: Which of the following is <u>NOT</u> a complication of the endobronchial balloon tamponade?

A. Vocal cords granulation tissue
B. Catheter migration
C. Lobar Pneumonia
D. Respiratory failure

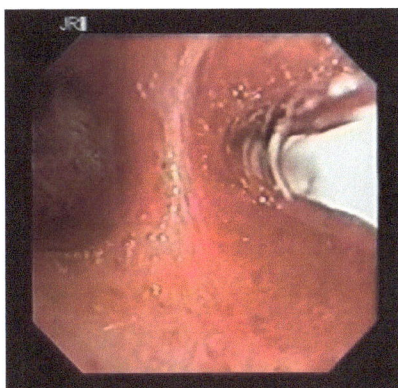

Answer II.13:   D

Management of airway bleeding depends on a structured yet flexible approach by a multidisciplinary team including anesthesia, thoracic surgery, interventional pulmonology, and interventional radiology (1). The strategy can be divided into 3 steps: stabilization, securing the airway and bleeding control. The choices of bleeding control include flexible or rigid bronchoscopy, endoluminal approaches, and surgery. One method for bleeding control is by tamponade, which can be achieved through several means. The most common way is by introducing an endobronchial blocker (usually used to facilitate single lung ventilation) through the endobronchial tube (ETT) itself, under bronchoscopic guidance. Another alternative is to introduce it through the cords alongside the endotracheal tube. Maneuvering the blocker alongside the ETT is more cumbersome than through the tube, and can irritate the vocal cords causing granulomas. An advantage, however, is leaving the endotracheal tube open for bronchoscopic evacuation of clots and other therapies. Large bronchial blockers can theoretically migrate in the trachea and cause respiratory failure, although to our knowledge there are no published reports of this complication.

Segmental bronchial bleeding can be stopped by tamponade with the use of a Fogarty catheter, a standard pulmonary artery catheter, or other specially designed catheters. If left in for a long time, necessary care should be taken to minimize the incidence of mucosal necrosis, such as inflating the balloon to the minimum and to deflate it periodically.

These tamponade devices can be left in for several days to facilitate more definitive therapy. However, post-obstructive pneumonia may develop during this time. Adverse effects of endobronchial balloon tamponade, therefore, include lobar pneumonia, transient hoarseness because of granulation tissue on the vocal cords, and catheter migration. Respiratory failure has not been reported as a complication of this procedure.

References

1. Yendamuri S. Massive Airway Hemorrhage. Thorac Surg Clin 2015; 25(3): 255-60.

Question II.14: A patient presented with massive hemoptysis from a right middle lobe abscess. A blood clot has formed in the RML bronchus after instillation of 200 ml of cold saline. The rest of the airways have been cleaned from hemorrhagic secretions. Patient's oxygenation is stable at 95% on facemask F_iO_2 0.3. Which of the following should be done next?

A. Remove the clot to restore right middle lobe bronchial patency.
B. Do not remove the clot and refer the patient to interventional radiology for bronchial artery embolization.
C. Selectively intubate the left main bronchus with an endotracheal tube.

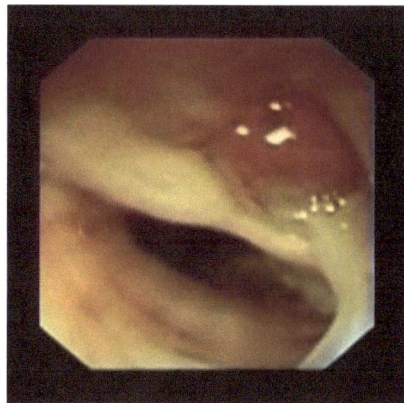

Answer II.14:   B

Immediate administration of large aliquots of iced saline using a wedged or partially wedged bronchoscope, continuous or intermittent suction, and gravity dependent clot formation stops most bleeding. Freshly formed clot should not be removed (1). Once clot forms, it is important to NOT remove it once bleeding has stopped. Inspection bronchoscopy (with or without clot removal) can be performed the following day. Large blood clot causes a cast of the distal airways (See Figure). Adverse effects on respiration, cardiac, and hemodynamic status should be avoided. Anxiolytics and narcotics have detrimental effects on respiration. In case of bleeding, additional intravenous sedation can result in adverse events such as respiratory failure, hypoxemia, and hypercapnia, hypotension and aspiration pneumonia. Reversing agents should be available. If additional sedation or anxiolysis is necessary, endotracheal intubation may be warranted even after bleeding is controlled. In this case, intubation with a large endotracheal tube should be considered. Intubation is usually possible with a large single lumen endotracheal tube inserted over the bronchoscope. Selective unilateral bronchial intubation is only possible if the oral route is used. A bite block to prevent patients from biting the bronchoscope (regardless of the level of sedation) should always be inserted prior to oral intubation over the bronchoscope.

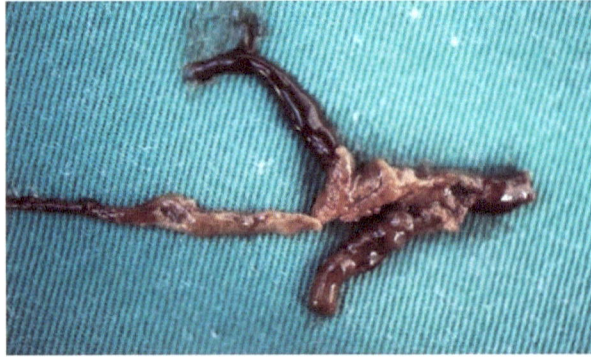

Bronchial cast with blood (Photo courtesy L. Oto)

References

1. Sakr L, Dutau H. Massive hemoptysis: an update on the role of bronchoscopy in diagnosis and management. Respiration 2010; 80(1): 38-58.

Question II.15: Most evidence for bronchoscopic management of massive hemoptysis is for:

A.   Instillation of Tranexamic acid
B.   Application of cold saline
C.   Balloon tamponade

Answer II.15:   C

While these three techniques are options for massive hemoptysis, most evidence is for balloon tamponade as illustrated in a review of the literature (1). Tranexamic Acid (TA) is an antifibrinolytic drug which is administered via the oral or intravenous route. It is widely used for the treatment or prophylaxis of mucosal bleeding in patients with bleeding disorders or following major surgery (1). Several case reports documenting its efficacy in controlling major hemoptysis in cystic fibrosis patients have been published. Topical administration of TA within the bronchial tree was described only recently. The first case of endobronchial irrigation with cold saline for the early management of hemoptysis was reported in 1980 (1). Lavage with normal saline at 4°C in 50-ml aliquots (average volume of 500 ml, range 300–750 ml) stopped the bleeding in 23 patients with massive hemoptysis (≥600 ml/24 h), obviating the need for emergency thoracotomy. A rigid bronchoscope was used during the session, and was introduced in an alternate manner on the nonbleeding side in order to isolate the lung and enable gas exchanges, and subsequently on the bleeding side to evacuate clots and large amounts of blood, as well as for local irrigation. One patient experienced transient sinus bradycardia during the procedure. Only 2 subjects suffered subsequent episodes of massive bleeding 3 and 10 days later. Both required further lavage.

The successful use of a Fogarty balloon catheter for endobronchial tamponade in life-threatening hemoptysis was initially described in 1974. It was inserted through a flexible fiber-optic bronchoscope in the right main bronchus, inflated and kept in place as an emergency measure in a hemodynamically unstable patient following bouts of severe hemoptysis. Freitag et al. developed a double-lumen bronchus-blocking balloon catheter, usually inserted into the working channel of a flexible bronchoscope (1). Kato et al. described a modified bronchoscopic balloon tamponade technique: an angiography J guide wire (0.035 in) is inserted through the working channel of a flexible bronchoscope, followed by removal of the bronchoscope and insertion of a balloon catheter (7 Fr) over the guide wire into a segmental bronchus (1). Another balloon tamponade technique uses a pulmonary artery balloon catheter. The catheter is introduced next to a flexible bronchoscope, guided through the endobronchial route, and inflated in segmental or subsegmental bronchi.

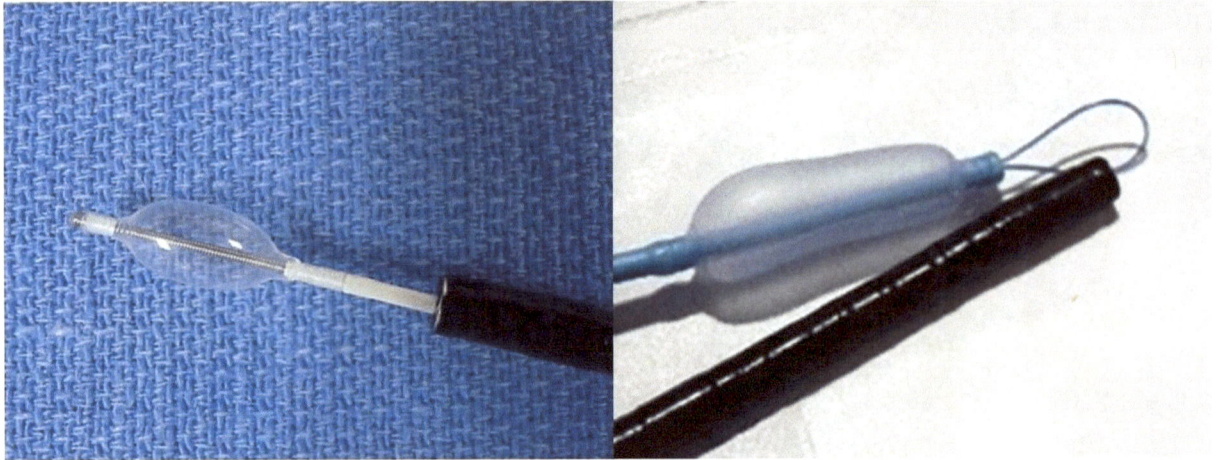

Examples of devices used for balloon tamponade

Left panel: Fogarty catheter can be inserted in a bleeding segmental bronchus; **Right panel:** Arndt endobronchial blocker can be inserted through or alongside an endotracheal tube. The blocker can be kept in place between 15 min and 1 week and is only deflated for a few minutes three times a day, in order to preserve mucosal viability and to check for bleeding recurrence.

References

2. Sakr L, Dutau H. Massive hemoptysis: an update on the role of bronchoscopy in diagnosis and management. Respiration 2010; 80(1): 38-58.

Question II.16: A patient is admitted to the Intensive Care Unit with recurrent hemoptysis and impending respiratory failure. Flexible bronchoscopy reveals a large, actively bleeding, tracheal tumor with destroyed cartilage obstructing most of the tracheal lumen. Which of the following interventional techniques is <u>least</u> suitable for restoring airway patency and controlling hemoptysis in this case?

A.   Laser photocoagulation
B.   Contact electrocautery
C.   Argon plasma coagulation
D.   Photodynamic therapy

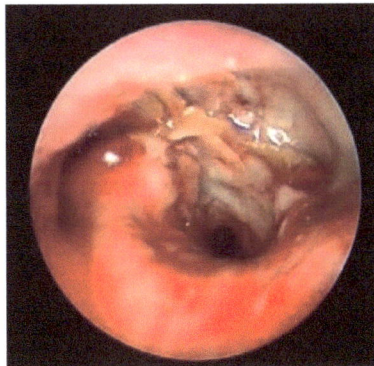

Answer II.16:   D

Nd: YAG laser coagulation is an effective treatment option for hemoptysis when the source of bleeding is bronchoscopically visible. Improvement in hemoptysis was noted in 94% of cancer patients who underwent endobronchial Nd: YAG laser treatment, with complete cessation of bleeding in 74% (1).

Argon plasma coagulation (APC) should be used only when the source of bleeding is within the reach of the bronchoscope as in the case of YAG laser photocoagulation. It provides easy access to lesions located laterally or around anatomic corners. In a retrospective study by Morice et al., 31 patients with hemoptysis (25 patients with concurrent airway obstruction) were treated by endobronchial APC therapy (1). Airway hemorrhage stopped immediately after the procedure in all patients with an endoluminal source of bleeding. No recurrence of bleeding was observed after a mean follow-up period of 97 days.

Contact Electrocautery to control hemoptysis can be used as well. In a study of 56 patients with advanced lung cancer or benign tumors, control of hemoptysis using endobronchial electrocautery was achieved in 75% of the cases (1).

Photodynamic therapy (PDT) can be used to facilitate minimally-invasive treatment of early endobronchial tumors and to palliate obstructive and bleeding effects of advanced endobronchial tumors (2). PDT is, however, a delayed effect therapy. The tumor cell death and necrosis occur approximately 48 hours after the illumination phase. Thus this is a suboptimal technique for emergent situations such as critical airway obstruction from a tumor or massive hemoptysis from endoluminal tumors.

References

1. Sakr L, Dutau H. Massive hemoptysis: an update on the role of bronchoscopy in diagnosis and management. Respiration 2010; 80(1): 38-58.
2. Kidane B, Hirpara D, Yasufuku K. Photodynamic Therapy in Non-Gastrointestinal Thoracic Malignancies. Int J Mol Sci 2016; 17(1). pii: E135.

Question II.17: Transbronchial lung biopsy is contraindicated in patients on mechanical ventilation because of high risk for bleeding and pneumothorax. This statement is:

A.   True
B.   False

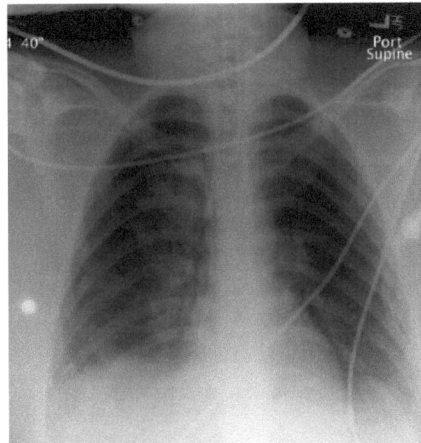

Answer II.17:   B

A transbronchial lung biopsy is not contraindicated, but risks should be carefully considered and the procedure should be performed only if results truly alter patient management. Bulpa et al. evaluated the safety and diagnostic yield of bronchoalveolar lavage (BAL) combined with transbronchial lung biopsy (TBLB) in determining the etiology of pulmonary infiltrates in mechanically ventilated patients (1). Patients were divided into two groups: immunocompetent (group 1 with and without ARDS) and immunocompromised (group 2). Positive end-expiratory pressure (PEEP) was maintained at ≤5 cmH$_2$O. Pneumothorax occurred in 23.6% (including 4/11 patients with ARDS), bleeding in 10.5% (<35 mL), and transient hypotension in 5% of the patients. No fatalities were procedure-related. No blood transfusion was needed. Subgroup analysis showed higher pneumothorax rate in late phase ARDS and bleeding if platelets were < 72,000.

In another study, twenty-five flexible bronchoscopic procedures with TBLB were performed in 24 severely thrombocytopenic immunocompromised patients (mean platelet count of 30,000/mm^3, range of 7,000/mm^3 to 60,000/mm^3) during the diagnostic evaluation of pulmonary infiltrates (2). Three patients had self-limited endobronchial bleeding. A single death was attributable to massive hemorrhage after transbronchial biopsy and brushing. Specific etiologic diagnoses were established by bronchoscopy in only nine cases.

References

1. Bulpa PA, Dive AM, Mertens L, Delos MA, Jamart J, Evrard PA, Gonzalez MR, Installé EJ. Combined bronchoalveolar lavage and transbronchial lung biopsy: safety and yield in ventilated patients. Eur Respir J 2003; 21(3): 489-94.
2. Papin TA, Lynch JP 3rd, Weg JG. Transbronchial biopsy in the thrombocytopenic patient. Chest 1985; 88(4): 549-52.

Question II.18: A 22-year-old man had a collision accident while snowboarding. He has an asymptomatic small pneumothorax on the initial chest CT. He is now on mechanical ventilation post op for fractured right humerus. What should be done next?

A.   Insert a 32 F chest tube via open thoracostomy
B.   Insert a 20 F chest tube by Seldinger technique
C.   Clinical and radiographic monitoring

Answer II.18:   C

Adults with traumatic occult pneumothoraces (OPTXs) (5% of all hospitalized trauma patients) and requiring positive-pressure ventilation (PPV) were randomized to pleural drainage or observation (1). The primary outcome was a composite of respiratory distress (RD) (need for urgent pleural drainage, acute/sustained increases in O2 requirements, ventilator desynchrony, and/or charted respiratory events). A total of 90 patients were enrolled (50 had chest tube; 40 observation). The risk of RD was similar between the observation and tube thoracostomy groups (relative risk, 0.71; 95% confidence interval, 0.40-1.27). There was no difference in mortality or intensive care unit (ICU), ventilator, or hospital days between groups. In those observed, 20% required subsequent pleural drainage (40% PTX progression, 60% pleural fluid, and 20% other). One observed patient (2%) undergoing PPV at enrollment had a tension PTX, which was treated with urgent tube thoracostomy without sequelae. Drainage complications occurred in 15% of those randomized to drainage, while suboptimal tube thoracostomy position occurred in an additional 15%. There were three times (24% vs. 8%) more failures and more RDs (p = 0.01) among those observed with OPTXs requiring sustained PPV versus just for an operation; this risk increases threefold after a week in the ICU (p = 0.07).

References

1. Kirkpatrick AW, Rizoli S, Ouellet JF, Roberts DJ, Sirois M, Ball CG, Xiao ZJ, Tiruta C, Meade M, Trottier V, Zhu G, Chagnon F, Tien H; Canadian Trauma Trials Collaborative and the Research Committee of the Trauma Association of Canada. Occult pneumothoraces in critical care: a prospective multicenter randomized controlled trial of pleural drainage for mechanically ventilated trauma patients with occult pneumothoraces. J Trauma Acute Care Surg 2013; 74(3): 747-54; discussion 754-5.

Question II.19: Evidence suggests that compared with low PEEP, the high PEEP ventilatory strategy in ARDS results in:

A.   Higher mortality and vasopressor requirement
B.   Higher incidence of pneumothorax
C.   More prolonged air leak post lung biopsy

Answer II.19:   C

One meta-analysis evaluated the impact on patient outcomes of higher vs. lower PEEP in adults with acute lung injury or ARDS who receive ventilation with low tidal volumes (1). Data from 2299 individual patients in 3 trials were analyzed using uniform outcome definitions. Both groups had low tidal volume ventilation. The mortality rate was 32.9% in higher PEEP group and 35.2% in the lower PEEP. Rates of pneumothorax and vasopressor use were similar. It was concluded that treatment with higher vs. lower levels of PEEP was not associated with improved hospital survival.

A retrospective study was done of 53 patients who underwent open lung biopsy for ARDS. Thirty percent of the patients developed an air leak lasting more than 7 days or died with an air leak (2). Persistent air leak (PAL) was inversely related to lower peak airway pressure, tidal volume and use of pressure-cycled ventilation. Peak airway pressure remained the significant predictor of PAL in multivariate analysis. The risk of PAL was reduced by 42% for every 5 cm H_2O reduction in peak airway pressure. It is noteworthy, that PEEP and peak inspiratory pressure are distinct and not always related.

References

1. Briel M, Meade M, Mercat A, Brower RG, Talmor D, Walter SD, Slutsky AS, Pullenayegum E, Zhou Q, Cook D, Brochard L, Richard JC, Lamontagne F, Bhatnagar N, Stewart TE, Guyatt G. Higher vs lower positive end-expiratory pressure in patients with acute lung injury and acute respiratory distress syndrome: systematic review and meta-analysis. JAMA 2010; 303(9): 865-73.
2. Cho MH, Malhotra A, Donahue DM, Wain JC, Harris RS, Karmpaliotis D, Patel SR. Mechanical ventilation and air leaks after lung biopsy for acute respiratory distress syndrome. Ann Thorac Surg 2006; 82(1): 261-6.

Question II.20: In case of massive hemoptysis the priority is to:

A.   Transfuse blood as soon as possible
B.   Establish and maintain an open airway
C.   Stop the bleeding

Answer II.20:   B

In managing patients with massive hemoptysis, the goals of treatment are to 1) establish and maintain an open airway; 2) stop the bleeding, and; 3) prevent or treat associated respiratory, cardiac, and hemodynamic compromise (1).

Maintaining an open airway in bleeding patients is possible by doing one or more of the following: 1) Bronchoscopic suction and large bore suction of the oral pharynx in non-intubated patients;2) Lateral safety position (bleeding side down, allows face to face contact with patient if operator working from the front or side of the patient, allows blood and secretions to flow from the larynx and out of the corner of the mouth, avoids collapse of the larynx and laryngeal obstruction by tongue or edematous upper airway, oral pharynx easily suctioned; turning the patient onto the "safety position" (bleeding side down) also protects the contra lateral airway in every patient with hemoptysis; 3) Note the bleeding site and remember how to get back to it as tamponade the bleeding bronchus using continuous bronchoscopic suction may suffice as in cases of bleeding post transbronchial biopsy; 4) Unilateral intubation may be needed when bleeding persists.

Bleeding is stopped using a variety of strategies: 1) Tamponade (Bronchoscopic suction, Balloons, the rigid bronchoscope, cotton pledgets, tampons) 2) Vasoconstriction agents (Epinephrine, cold saline washes, Intravenous vasopressin (0.2 - 0.4 units / min) causes bronchial arterial vasoconstriction: epinephrine and vasopressin are not favored if patient has coronary artery disease and hypertension; in addition, there are reports of tachyarrhythmias with these agents, and there is no scientific evidence that epinephrine is better than iced saline. washes ; 3) Enhance clot formation (Allow clot to form in the bleeding area, Lateral decubitus position). If a tamponade balloon or Fogarty catheter is inserted into a bleeding segmental bronchus, its position should be verified by flexible bronchoscopy and chest radiograph. The balloon can remain in place for several days if necessary. Tamponade balloons or dilating balloons should be large enough to tamponade a bleeding segmental and subsegmental airway. A Fogarty balloon catheter can be used but operators and their assistants should first verify that balloon diameter is sufficient to fill segmental bronchial airway and that balloon catheter fits through working channel of the bronchoscope. The Cook (Arndt) bronchial blocker, if necessary, should be inserted through a large endotracheal tube (ETT), or alongside a regular size ETT. The catheter can be kept in place between 15 min and 1 week and is only deflated for a few minutes 3 times a day, in order to preserve mucosal viability and to check for bleeding recurrence.

Respiratory, cardiac, and hemodynamic instability occur in patients with massive hemoptysis. Blood transfusion and endotracheal intubation may be necessary and should be initiated early on in the management algorithm. Blood clots also can cause airway obstruction, hypoxemia, and death, so decision-making includes whether or not to remove clots and to perform bronchoscopic airway inspection frequently if needed. Morbidity related to airway bleeding is explained on the basis of physiologic consequences of airway bleeding: blood filling of dead-space (anatomic dead space= 150 ml), airway obstruction and clot formation, subsequent tachypnea and hypoxemia, tachycardia, bradycardia, hypotension, respiratory failure, arrhythmia and cardiac arrest. Underlying disease state (e.g. history of pneumonectomy, critically illness and significant comorbidities) is also very important as respiratory failure may develop even without a large amount of bleeding. Mortality rates from massive hemoptysis have ranged from 9 to 38%. Bronchovascular fistula is a rare disease mostly seen in the patients with lung transplant-related airway anastomotic ischemic or infectious necrosis, Rasmussen's aneurysms, transbronchial lung biopsy, endobronchial brachytherapy/photodynamic therapy, radiofrequency ablation or cancer.

Poor prognosticators of massive hemoptysis are bleeding rate of at least 1,000 ml within a 24-hour, aspiration of blood in the contralateral lung, massive bleeding requiring single-lung ventilation, lung cancer and recurrent bleeding following bronchial artery embolization (BAE).

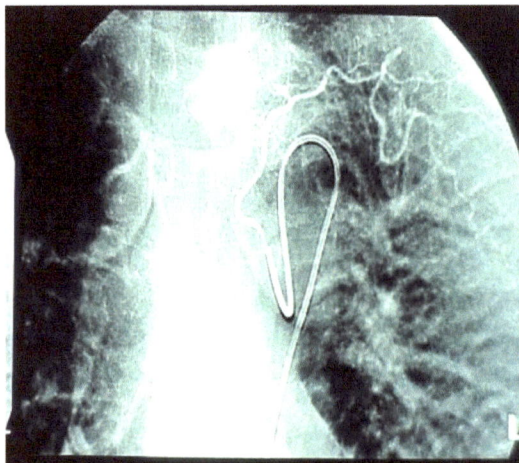

Bronchial embolization Left Upper Lobe T5 level

References

(1). Sakr L, Dutau H. Massive hemoptysis: an update on the role of bronchoscopy in diagnosis and management. Respiration 2010; 80(1): 38-58.

Question II.21: A 50-year-old male with a remote history of chest trauma and respiratory failure requiring intubation and two weeks of mechanical ventilation develops wheezing and dyspnea shortly after extubation. Physical examination reveals decreased breath sounds on the right and audible wheezing. Flexible bronchoscopy reveals the image below. The most likely diagnosis:

A.   Ventilator-associated tracheitis
B.   Rhinoscleroma
C.   Aspergillus tracheitis
D.   Tuberculous tracheitis

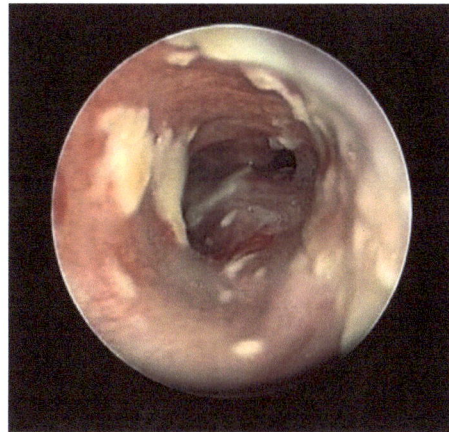

Answer II.21:   A

Ventilator-associated tracheitis may be seen in an immunocompromised host on cephalosporins and can cause central airway obstruction. Appropriate antibiotics are used and sometimes tracheostomy is recommended. Obstructive bacterial tracheobronchitis is rare. *Staphylococcus aureus* is the most commonly implicated bacterial organism, isolated from the respiratory tract in 55.8% of the cases with bacterial tracheitis (1). MRSA necrotizing tracheitis can be fulminant (2).

Other infectious causes of tracheitis, however, can also present with a similar pattern. For example, Tuberculosis tracheitis can have an actively caseating, edematous-hyperemic, fibrostenotic, appearance. Such an actively caseating type (43.0%) is the most common form and is highly contagious (See Figure below) (3, 4).

Aspergillus can have various appearances, including similar to the photo above. Thick, raised, white plaque-like forms can sometimes be peeled off airway mucosa, prompting minor bleeding of the mucosa beneath (5).

Klebsiella Rhinoscleroma, a subspecies of Klebsiella pneumonia has a special affinity for the nasal mucosa may also cause upper airway obstruction. It may be limited to nasal passages but laryngeal involvement is seen in 15-80% and the recurrence rate is up to 25% over 10 years of follow up (6).

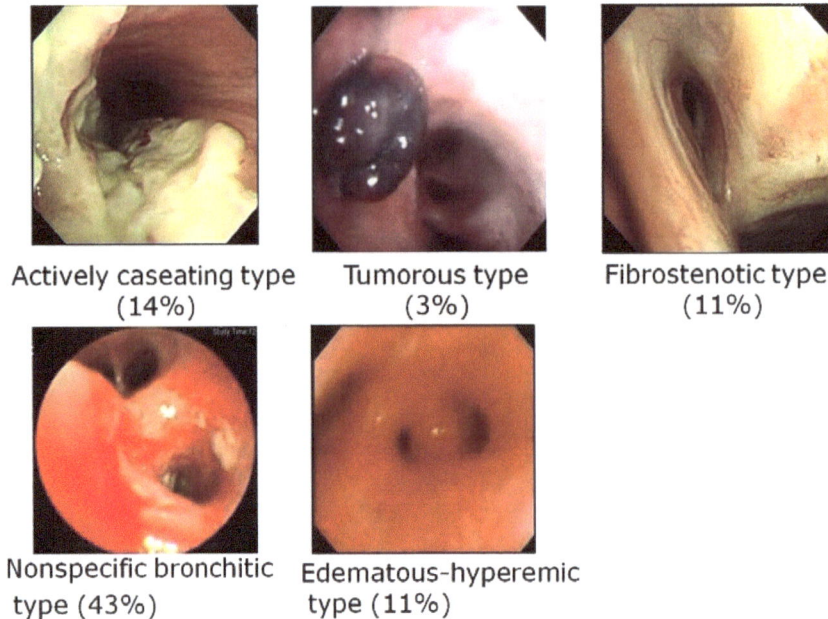

Actively caseating type (14%)   Tumorous type (3%)   Fibrostenotic type (11%)

Nonspecific bronchitic type (43%)   Edematous-hyperemic type (11%)

Forms of endobronchial tuberculosis (percentages as per Chung and Lee, Chest 2000)

References

1. Tebruegge M, Pantazidou A, Thorburn K, Riordan A, Round J, De Munter C, Walters S, Curtis N. Bacterial tracheitis: a multi-center perspective. Scand J Infect Dis 2009; 41(8): 548-57.
2. Namba Y, Mihara N, Tanaka M. [Fulminant tracheobronchitis caused by methicillin-resistant Staphylococcus aureus (MRSA)]. Nihon Kyobu Shikkan Gakkai Zasshi 1997; 35(9): 969-73.
3. Chung HS, Lee JH. Bronchoscopic assessment of the evolution of endobronchial tuberculosis. Chest 2000; 117(2): 385-92.
4. Chung HS. Endobronchial tuberculosis. From Tuberculosis, pages 328-348, M Madkour, Eds. Springer-Verlag, Berlin 2003.
5. Karnak D, Avery RK, Gildea TR, Sahoo D, Mehta AC. Endobronchial fungal disease: an under-recognized entity. Respiration 2007; 74(1): 88-104.
6. Gaafar HA, Gaafar AH, Nour YA. Rhinoscleroma: an updated experience through the last 10 years. Acta Otolaryngol 2011; 131(4): 440-6.

Question II.22: The CT scan image below is from a patient with hemoptysis. During his first night in the Intensive Care Unit, he expectorated a total of 150 cc of bright red blood and sputum into a cup. This amount of hemoptysis might be classified as:

A.   Moderate hemoptysis
B.   Severe hemoptysis
C.   Major hemoptysis
D.   Massive hemoptysis

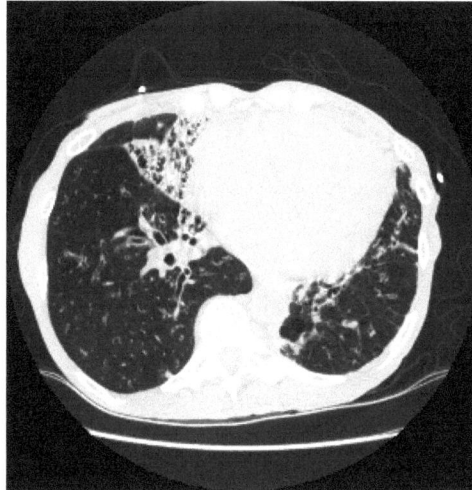

Answer II.22:   B

The volume of expectorated blood has often been used to define episodes of hemoptysis. Amounts of expectorated blood ranging from 100 ml/24 h to more than 1,000 ml/24 h have been proposed to define "massive hemoptysis". Other terms, such as 'major' hemoptysis (≥200 ml/24 h), severe hemoptysis (≥150 ml/12 h and >400 ml/24 h) and 'exsanguinating hemoptysis' (≥1,000 ml total or ≥150 ml/h) are also employed to describe the extent of bleeding. The difficulty, of course, in quantifying hemoptysis is that often blood is mixed in with sputum. Regardless, bleeding of any sort is extremely anxiety-provoking for both patients and doctors. Any bleed may represent a sentinel event signaling a life-threatening subsequent episode, and therefore should be taken very seriously. Observation in the ICU is usually warranted, keeping an endotracheal tube at the bedside, and informing the airway emergency team, anesthesiology, and thoracic surgery of the patient's admission.

A CT scan will often detect the site of bleeding and may precede attempts at embolization if indicated. Bleeding usually originates from the high-pressure bronchial circulation (90%). Pulmonary arteries remain the source of bleeding in a number of patients

(5%) usually suffering from necrotizing pulmonary infections, pulmonary abscess, cavitary lung carcinoma, Hodgkin's lymphoma, vasculitis, trauma from a pulmonary artery (Swan-Ganz) catheter and pulmonary arteriovenous malformation.

Question II.23: A patient with squamous cell bronchogenic carcinoma is admitted to the intensive care unit with impending respiratory failure (see chest radiograph below) Which of the following statements regarding malignant central airway obstruction is correct?

A. Successful palliation is highly dependent on the type of bronchoscopic method used to restore airway potency.
B. Despite restored central airway patency, the majority of patients with malignant obstruction die within 30 days.
C. ICU admission and referral for possible bronchoscopic intervention is justified in most patients with malignant central airway obstruction.

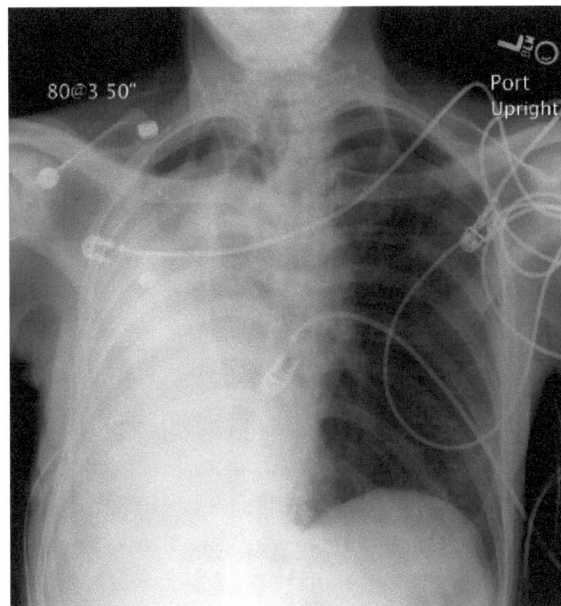

Answer II.23   C

    High-dose-rate brachytherapy (HDR) alone, HDR plus Nd: YAG, stent insertion, Nd:YAG alone and photodynamic therapy (PDT) alone were reviewed to determine the most effective management strategy for inoperable malignant airway obstruction in another study (1). The majority of patients managed with HDR, Nd:YAG, or HDR plus Nd:YAG received good to excellent short-term palliation, suggesting that restoring airway potency leads to improved outcomes, likely independent of the modality used. In another study, intubated patients with respiratory failure caused by central airway obstruction (CAO) from NSCLC were successfully and rapidly removed from mechanical ventilation after bronchoscopic interventions aimed at restoring airway patency (2). Median survival greater than 10 months justifies ICU admission and referral for bronchoscopic intervention (the chest radiograph below shows lung reexpansion after removal of right-sided central airway obstruction)

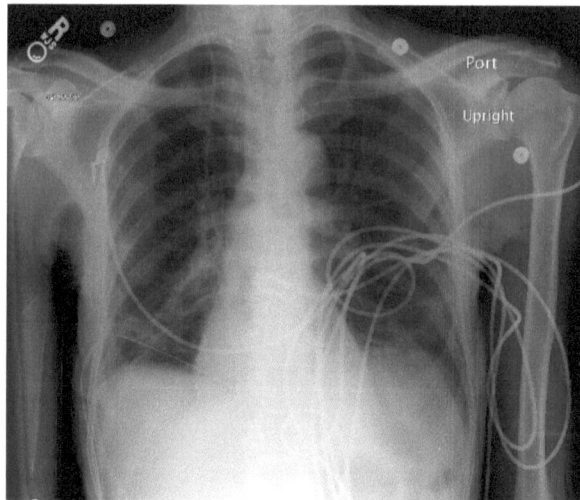

References

1. Morris CD, Budde JM, Godette KD, Kerwin TL, Miller JI Jr. Palliative management of malignant airway obstruction. Ann Thorac Surg 2002; 74(6): 1928-32; discussion 1932-3.
2. Murgu S, Langer S, Colt H. Bronchoscopic intervention obviates the need for continued mechanical ventilation in patients with airway obstruction and respiratory failure from inoperable non-small-cell lung cancer. Respiration 2012; 84(1): 55-61.

Question II.24 The following image is most consistent with:

A. Granulomatosis with polyangiitis (GPA) formerly known as Wegener's.
B. Tracheal Amyloidosis
C. Sarcoidosis

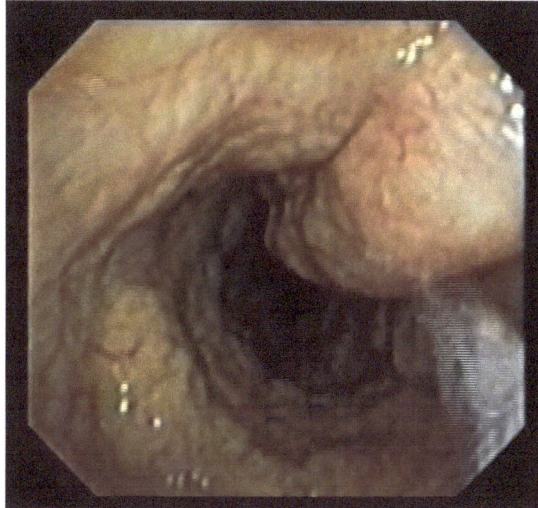

Answer II.24   B

Amyloidosis is caused by over expression and extracellular deposition of specific proteins (1). Tracheobronchial amyloidosis is a rare disorder characterized by airway deposition of amyloid material as submucosal plaques and/or polypoid tumors. There are two forms of airway amyloidosis: a nodular or unifocal disease and a diffuse submucosal disease. Airway involvement in amyloidosis is seen with the AL type in which the specific protein deposition is comprised of kappa and lambda light chains of monoclonal immunoglobulins. Treatment of the airway disease includes low dose EBRT (20 Gy in 10 fractions) and frequent laser resections (~ 5/ year).

Granulomatosis with polyangiitis (GPA), formerly referred to as Wegener's granulomatosis (WG), involves the airways in approximately 60% of the patients (2). Subglottic stenosis is seen in 16% of the patients with GPA; ~60% of pts with limited disease are ANCA positive. Intralesional steroids and Mitomycin C are used for treatment. GPA, independent of other features of disease activity may be associated subglottic strictures. Subglottic stenosis may be the presenting feature in 1-6% of patients; 75-80% of patients require interventional bronchoscopy because they do not respond to steroid therapy. Multiple bronchoscopic dilations with minimal trauma and managing of inflammation are the main treatment strategies. The 10-year survival is 75%. Bronchoscopic findings may also include submucosal tunnels, mucosa edema, erythema and yellow mucosal plaques that are easily confused with localized amyloidosis. Bronchial stenosis can be bilateral. Some airway narrowing may persist (with or without residual inflammation) even months after bronchoscopic treatment (see Figure below).

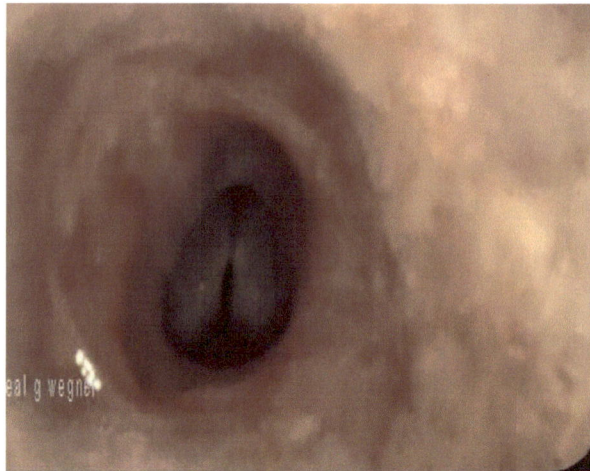

Example of residual subglottic stricture after bronchoscopic treatment in a 29-year-old female with GPA. Scope inserted through tracheostomy, vocal cords are seen from below.

References

1. Lebovics RS, Hoffman GS, Leavitt RY, et al. The management of subglottic stenosis in patients with Wegener's granulomatosis. Laryngoscope 1992; 102:1341-1345.
2. Kurrus JA, Hayes JK, Hoidal JR, et al. Radiation therapy for tracheobronchial amyloidosis. Chest 1998; 114(5): 1489-1492.

Question II.25 A 45-year-old patient is admitted with increasing shortness of breath and a widened mediastinum on chest radiograph. Computer tomography scan reveals bilateral lymphadenopathy and a widened subcarina. Physical examination reveals occasional wheezing. The patient is a cigarette smoker and has a family history of early lung cancer (his father died at age 50, mother died at age 48, each from bronchogenic carcinoma). The patient is hospitalized overnight in the intensive care unit and referred for inspection bronchoscopy and EBUS-TBNA the next morning. Based on the image below, which of the following is the most likely diagnosis?

A. Sarcoidosis
A. Metastatic prostate cancer
B. Bronchogenic carcinoma with mediastinal lymph node involvement

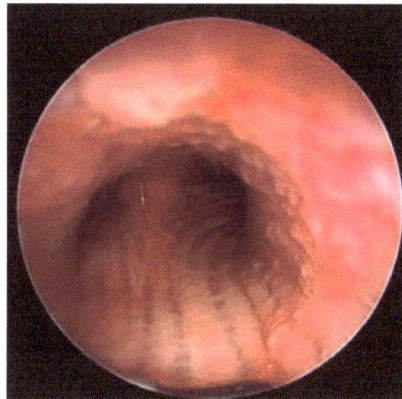

Answer II.25:   A

Sarcoidosis is a systemic granulomatous disease of unknown origin that commonly affects the bronchial tree (1). In stage 4 sarcoidosis, bronchial involvement often leads to bronchial narrowing by endobronchial and/or peribronchial fibrotic lesions; or by extrinsic compression by fibrotic and calcified lymph nodes. In stage 1–3 sarcoidosis, the mechanisms leading to endoluminal stenosis of proximal bronchi are different. Of a cohort of 2,500 patients with sarcoidosis, only 18 patients had bronchial stenosis (1). Cough was the main symptom. The bronchial mucosa appeared thickened, edematous and inflamed at the site of the stenosis in all cases. The mucosa outside the stenosis was inflamed in all patients, with fine granulations and nodules in 50% of patients. Tracheal stenosis due to sarcoidosis is extremely rare. Enlargement of the carina due to extrinsic compression by lymphadenopathy has been reported. Laryngeal sarcoidosis is estimated to be seen in 1.2% of patients suffering from this disease. It has been traditionally treated with systemic and intralesional injections of a corticosteroid, surgical intervention, carbon dioxide laser ablation, and even external beam radiation.

References

1. Chambellan A, Turbie P, Nunes H, Brauner M, Battesti JP, Valeyre D. Endoluminal stenosis of proximal bronchi in sarcoidosis: bronchoscopy, function, and evolution. Chest 2005; 127(2): 472-81.

Question II.26: Which of the following statements about iatrogenic pneumothorax in the ICU is correct?

A. Iatrogenic pneumothorax may be expected in up to 3 percent of ICU patients in their first 30 days of hospitalization.
B. Mortality rates for critically ill patients with iatrogenic pneumothorax in the ICU are less than 10 percent.
C. Morbid obesity is a known risk factor for iatrogenic pneumothorax.

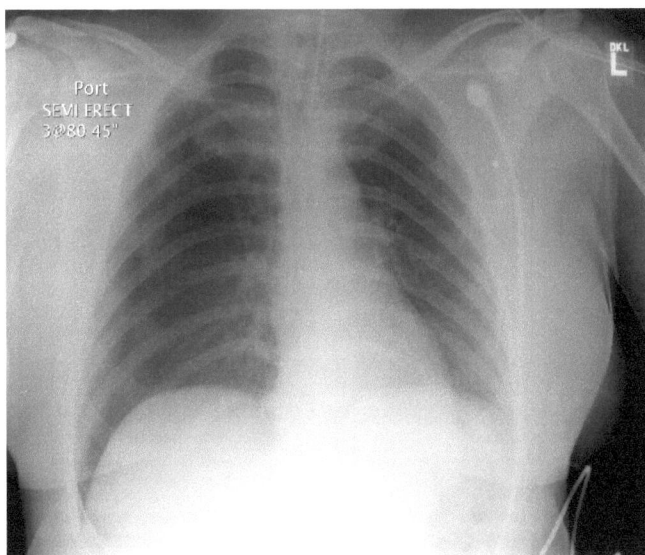

Answer II.26:   A

The incidence, risk factors, morbidity, and mortality of Iatrogenic pneumothorax (IP) were investigated in a prospective study including 3,430 patients (1). Among these, 94 (2.7%) patients experienced at least one episode of pneumothorax within the first 30 days (42 due to barotrauma and 52 due to invasive procedures). The cumulative incidence of IP was 1.4% on day 5 and 3.0% on day 30. Risk factors for iatrogenic pneumothorax were body weight less than 80 kg, history of adult immunodeficiency syndrome, diagnosis of cardiogenic pulmonary edema at admission, diagnosis of ARDS at admission, insertion of a central vein catheter or pulmonary artery catheter during the first 24 h of ICU stay, and use of vasoactive agents during the first 24 hours. Iatrogenic pneumothorax was associated with longer durations of the ICU stay (7 vs. 17.5 days) and hospital stay (18 vs. 31 days). Mortality rates in the ICU (22 vs. 45%) and hospital (28 vs. 51%) were also higher in patients with iatrogenic pneumothorax. It is noteworthy that ten of the 94 patients with iatrogenic pneumothorax died on the same day or the day after the event. Tension IP caused cardiac arrest in 10 patients (10.6%).

References

1. de Lassence A, Timsit JF, Tafflet M, Azoulay E, Jamali S, Vincent F, Cohen Y, Garrouste-Orgeas M, Alberti C, Dreyfuss D; OUTCOMEREA Study Group. Pneumothorax in the intensive care unit: incidence, risk factors, and outcome. Anesthesiology 2006; 104(1): 5-13.

Question II.27: The damage to the flexible bronchoscope in the Figure below most likely occurred in which of the following situations?

A. When the bronchoscope was placed into the scope washer
B. When the bronchoscope was placed into its storage case
C. When the bronchoscope was inserted orally through an endotracheal tube in a patient without the protection of a bite block.

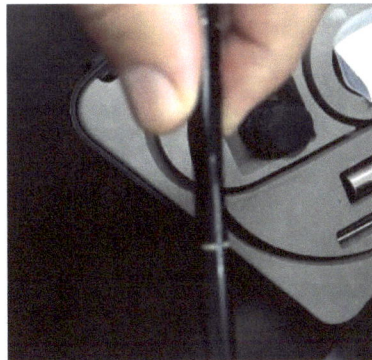

Answer II.27:   C

It can be quite embarrassing to discover that your patient has bitten down on your flexible bronchoscope, which is what is shown in the figure above. This occurs frequently when bronchoscopy is performed orally without the protection of a bite block. Bite blocks or other oral airways should always be placed when bronchoscopy is performed using the oral approach, even when patients are sedated. Bite blocks should be fixed into place using a neck strap, and ideally, an assistant may be asked to hold the bite block firmly in place as an additional precaution. Patients may inadvertently, or intentionally push the bite block out using their tongue, or remove it using their hands, or during a cough. Damage such as that shown in the figure also occurs when scopes are slammed inside drawers or against a procedure cart. Even more embarrassing is scope damage by closing the lid of a bronchoscope storage case on a scope that has not been properly placed within the protective foam covering of the case.

Question II.28: Flexible bronchoscopy is performed in a potential lung donor (multiple injuries from blunt trauma and brain death after an automobile accident) as part of lung transplant evaluation. The chest radiograph and bronchoscopic image below might prompt which of the following steps?

A. Tell the transplant team they may proceed with lung retrieval and subsequent transplant of both donor lungs.
B. Proceed with bronchial washing and send specimens for microbiology, including fungal and Acid-fast organisms. Inform the transplant team of the findings.
C. Request a computed tomography scan to evaluate the extent of abnormalities and obtain bronchial washings. Send washings for microbiology including fungal and acid-fast organisms.

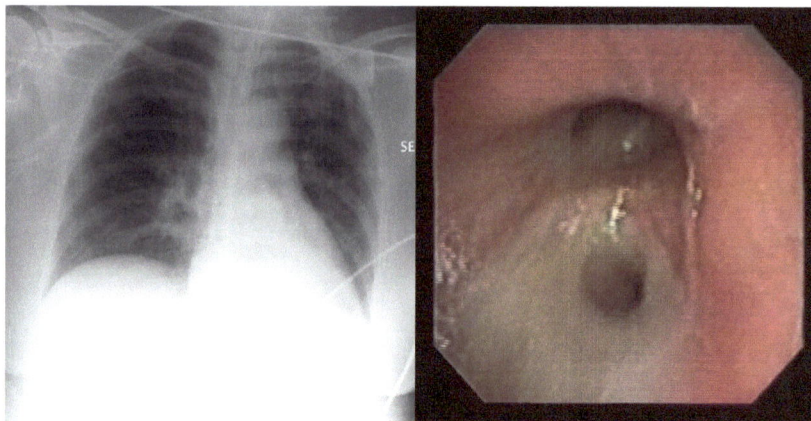

Pretransplant evaluation: Donor lungs

Answer II.28:   C

The chest radiograph has a relatively low sensitivity compared with computed tomography scans in the detection of lung abnormalities in potential lung donors, although lung scans are not considered routine as part of the donor lung evaluation by most transplant teams (1). Scans are probably warranted in donors with a history of smoking (to exclude lung malignancy or if emphysema is a concern), in donors with a history of penetrating trauma to evaluate the extent of lung contusions and exclude diaphragmatic tears or lung lacerations, in donors with a history of aspiration or lobar consolidation, and in patients over the age of 70 (because of the increased frequency of lung pathology).

Indications for bronchoscopy in potential lung donors include radiographic evidence of segmental or lobar collapse, significant secretions on endotracheal tube suctioning, assessment of pulmonary infiltrates (especially if unilateral), a history of aspiration, foreign body inhalation, or airway trauma, or endobronchial disease. Bronchoscopy is also performed in donors with unexpectedly low PO2, Bronchoscopy may be abnormal in up to 50% of potential lung donors. Abnormalities include mucus, blood clots, purulent bronchial secretions, and endobronchial abnormalities such as mass or findings consistent with infection or endobronchial disease. During the procedure, samples are obtained that might enhance antibiotic regimen selection post-transplantation. In addition to verifying the location of the indwelling endotracheal tube, bronchoscopists should examine airway anatomy searching for variations (particularly a right upper lobe tracheal bronchus),   evaluate extent of airway inflammation, edema or erythema, note the site and extent of secretions, foreign bodies, blood clots, tumors, or other endobronchial abnormalities. Secretions are aspirated, and washings are performed using small volume (5-20 cc) aliquots of saline solution. Specimens are sent to the microbiology laboratory for analysis, including fungal and Acid-fast bacteria stains.

References

1. Guidelines for lung donor bronchoscopy and CT Chest. ATCA-TSANZ Guidelines, 1/2015. Version 1.0.

Question II.29: During a respiratory emergency with difficult and partially blind intubation, the bronchoscope is inserted via the mouth and the following image is seen. The best course of action is to:

A. Proceed with intubation over the bronchoscope. Begin ventilation with an Ambu bag and secure the position of the endotracheal tube.
B. Inform the team of an esophageal/ gastric intubation. Quickly remove the bronchoscope and repeat the intubation attempt.
C. Remove the bronchoscope slowly under visual guidance in order to clearly see the larynx and vocal cords during removal. Insert the scope and endotracheal between the cords into the trachea.

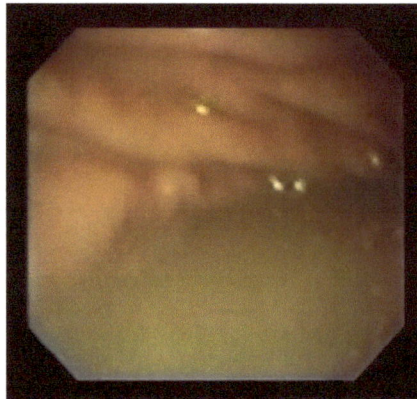

Answer II.29:   C

The image shows that the bronchoscope is not in the trachea. Gastric folds are seen as are gastric juices. Because there was difficulty visualizing airway anatomy (partially blind intubation), the scope should be removed slowly. If necessary, air can be insufflated via the accessory channel of the bronchoscope in order to prevent the collapse of the esophageal wall and larynx upon removal. As the scope is removed from the upper esophageal sphincter, it should be flexed slightly anterior in order to visualize the arytenoids and glottis aperture (vocal folds). The scope can then be immediately advanced into the trachea and the endotracheal tube guided over the flexible scope into the airway.

Question II.30: You have successfully performed an emergency intubation over the bronchoscope in the trauma holding area prior to moving the patient to the Intensive Care Unit. The patient's portable chest radiograph is shown below. Which of the following steps is most appropriate?

A. Repeat flexible bronchoscopy through the endotracheal tube and position the tube securely above the carina under direct visualization. Simultaneously, the team should prepare for chest tube insertion in view of the patient's left-sided pneumothorax.
B. Unsecure the endotracheal tube and pull it back at least two centimeters so it is in a more satisfactory position in the tracheal. Resecure the endotracheal tube and obtain a chest radiograph to confirm placement.
C. Proceed with mechanical ventilation and initiate an emergency transfer to the ICU after assuring that the patient's oxygenation is satisfactory. Prepare for left chest tube insertion in the ICU.

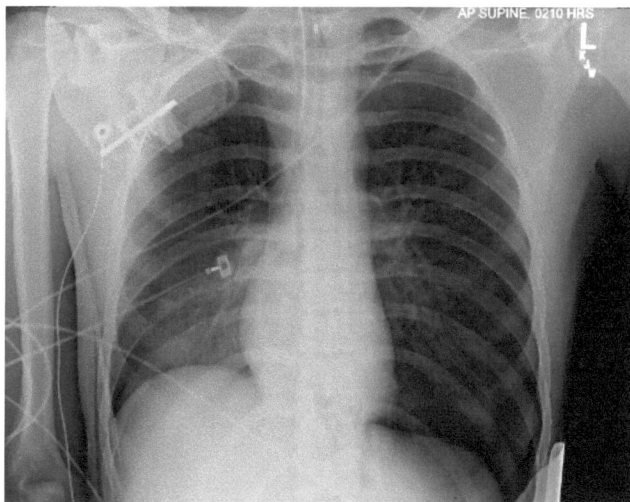

Answer II.30:   A

After emergency procedures such as intubation, even when done over the flexible bronchoscope, it is always necessary to carefully review the post-procedure chest radiograph to assure the endotracheal tube is in a satisfactory position, and to detect any new findings. This patient has a left-sided pneumothorax that will probably require drainage because the patient is on mechanical ventilation. In most instances, it is best to stabilize the patient prior to initiating the transfer, especially since increasing barotrauma may prompt further cardiopulmonary compromise (or tension pneumothorax) while the patient is being ventilated (by hand or machine) during transfer to the ICU.

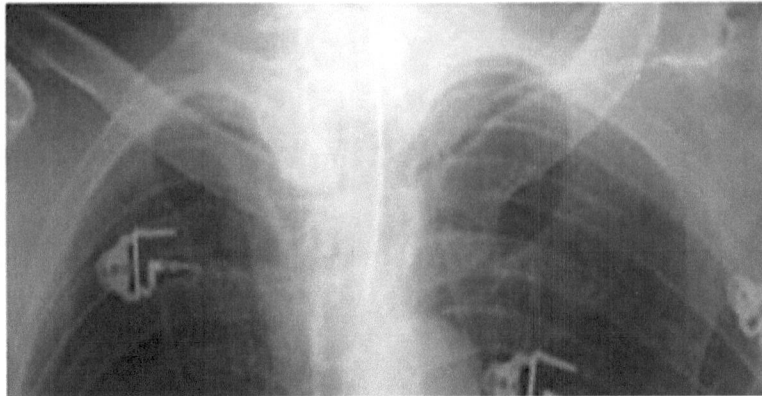

ET tube in higher position above carina.

***

CONGRATULATIONS

You have now completed Module II of The Essential Intensivist Bronchoscopist©.

The following section contains a ten-question post-test and answers.

Post-tests are True/False. Please remember that while many programs consider 70% correct responses a passing grade, the student's "target" score should be 100%.

Please send us your opinion regarding Bronchoscopy Education Project materials by contacting your national bronchology association or emailing us at
www.bronchoscopy.org.

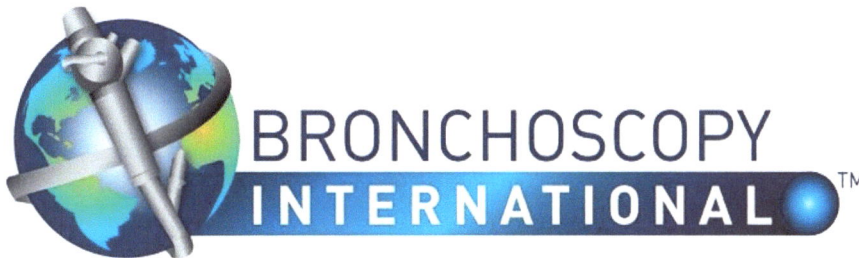

MODULE II

TEN QUESTION TRUE/FALSE POST-TEST

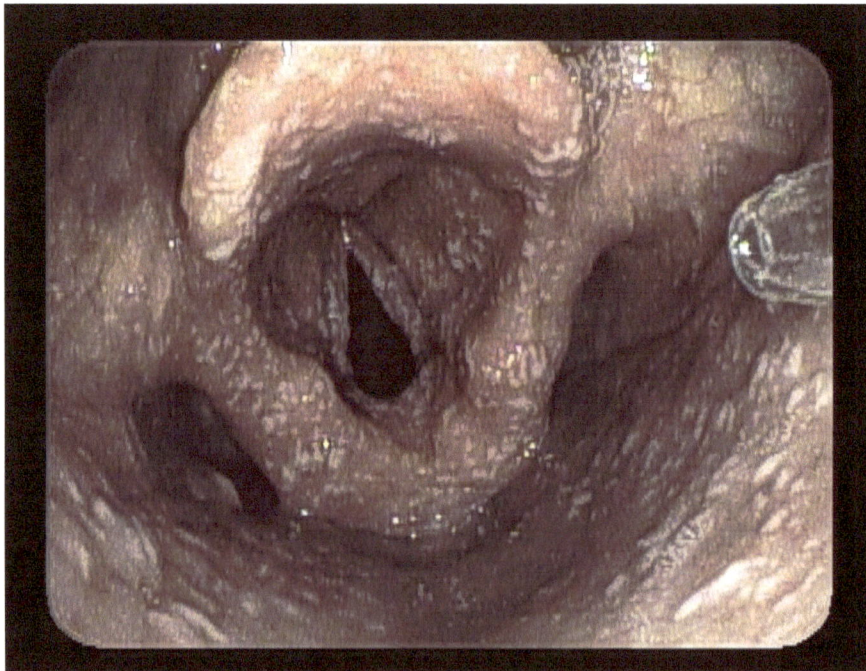

The Essential Intensivist Bronchoscopist

Module II Post-test

INSTRUCTIONS: Answer True or False to each of the following <u>TEN</u> questions.

Question 1: Non-invasive positive pressure ventilation (NPPV) improves lung mechanics and oxygenation in patients with hypoxemia.

Question 2: Early bronchoscopy favorably affects mortality and length of stay in the intensive care unit for intubated patients with possible aspiration pneumonia.

Question 3: Results from quantitative cultures obtained from bronchoalveolar lavage fluid in patients with ventilator-associated pneumonia favorably affect mortality and length of ICU stay.

Question 4: Bronchoscopy is better than chest physical therapy at resolving lobar atelectasis in critically ill patients.

Question 5: Therapeutic interventional bronchoscopy has little effect on length of stay or mortality in patients with malignant central airway obstruction.

Question 6: Actively caseating tuberculosis is the most frequent form of endobronchial tuberculosis and more than 50% of patients are acid-fast bacilli (AFB) smear-positive.

Question 7: A bite block should always be used to protect the flexible bronchoscope inserted through an oral endotracheal tube, even in fully sedated patients.

Question 8: The likelihood of detecting the site of bleeding is enhanced after early versus late bronchoscopy in patients with hemoptysis.

Question 9: Hypoxemia and exsanguination are the most frequent causes of death in patients with massive hemoptysis.

Question 10: Necrotizing tracheitis is a known complication of intubation and mechanical ventilation. Bronchoscopy with cultures is necessary to differentiate various forms of infection.

***

Answers to

The Essential Intensivist Bronchoscopist post-test Module II

ANSWERS

1. True
2. True
3. False
4. False
5. False
6. True
7. True
8. True
9. False
10. True

TOTAL SCORE _____/10

MODULE III

THIRTY MULTIPLE CHOICE QUESTION/ANSWER SETS

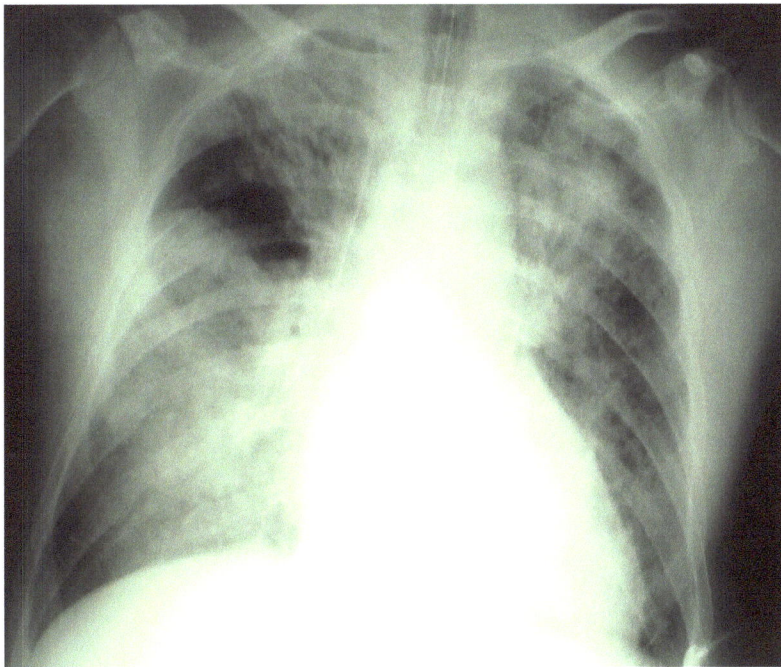

The Essential Intensivist Bronchoscopist©

The Essential Intensivist Bronchoscopist MODULE III

LEARNING OBJECTIVES

After completing this module the reader should be able to:

1. Mention diagnostic bronchoscopic strategies in patients with febrile neutropenia.
2. Describe the results of at least three bronchoscopy tests used to diagnose fungal pneumonia in critically ill patients.
3. List the Bronchoalveolar lavage findings in cases of ARDS imitators, including patients with diffuse alveolar hemorrhage, acute eosinophilic pneumonia, and acute idiopathic pneumonitis.
4. Describe the role of bronchoscopy in ICU patients with HIV infection, aspiration pneumonia, post lung transplant, burn injury and chest trauma.
5. List at least three diagnostic and preventive strategies for bronchoscopy-related complications that might lead to ICU admission (including oversedation, lidocaine toxicity, bleeding, methemoglobinemia and cerebral air embolism).
6. Describe the advantages and disadvantages of at least three pharmacologic agents used for sedation and/or anesthesia in patients undergoing bronchoscopy in the intensive care unit.

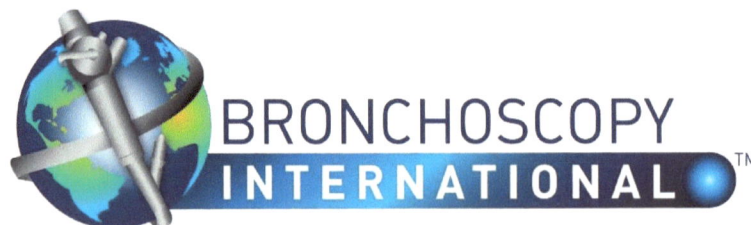

BRONCHOSCOPY INTERNATIONAL™

Question III.1: A patient with febrile neutropenia on chemotherapy for actual lymphocytic pneumonia presents with fever and hypoxemia requiring FiO_2 of 0.5 via facemask. The patient was admitted to the intensive care unit. The chest computed tomography shows bilateral lung infiltrates with nodular pattern and several peripheral, cavitary nodules. A few nodules have the "halo sign". Invasive aspergillosis (IPA) is suspected and the Infectious disease service requests a consult for a diagnostic bronchoscopy. Which of the following tests has the highest sensitivity and safety profile for diagnosing IPA?

A.   Bronchoalveolar lavage (BAL) galactomannan (GM) antigen
B.   Bronchoscopy with transbronchial lung biopsy (TBLB)
C.   Bronchoalveolar lavage (BAL) fungal stain and culture
D.   Serum galactomannan (GM) antigen

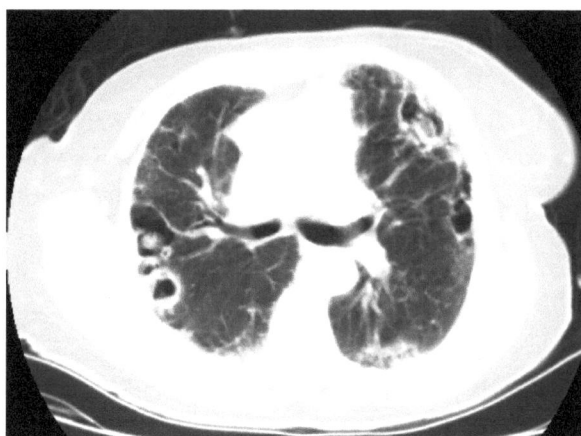

Answer III.1:   A

The favorable safety record, good diagnostic yield, and frequent therapeutic implications support the routine use of BAL for the evaluation of pulmonary infiltrates in neutropenic patients. BAL should be combined with the analysis of several sputum specimens, but TBLB adds little value in this patient population.

TBLB for IPA in patients who are immunocompromised may be avoided if BAL GM test is available due to the high sensitivity and specificity of the latter and inherent risk of biopsies. In one study, the effectiveness of BAL GM in diagnosing IPA was evaluated retrospectively (1). Using BAL GM ≥ 0.5 (cutoff for serum level) and ≥ 0.85 (optimal cutoff as determined by ROC analysis), the sensitivity in diagnosing proven or probable IPA was 73% and 67%, respectively, and specificity was 89% and 95%, respectively. Positive and negative predictive values were 73% and 83% (0.5); 89% and 87% (for 0.85), respectively.

BAL GM was more sensitive than cytology (0%), BAL culture (27%), TBLB (40%), or serum GM (67%) for diagnosing IPA. BAL GM was ≥ 0.85 and ≥ 0.5 in 86% and 100% of patients with proven or probable IPA who received an antifungal agent for ≤ 3 days. Thus, the sooner the bronchoscopy is performed, the higher the yield of the procedure. Furthermore, BAL GM added sensitivity to serum GM and other bronchoscopic techniques of diagnosing IPA and was not impacted by short courses of antifungal agents (1).

The safety, diagnostic yield, and therapeutic implications of flexible bronchoscopy with BAL and TBLB in patients with febrile neutropenia and pulmonary infiltrates were evaluated in another study (2). The overall diagnostic yield of BAL was 49%. The combined diagnostic yield of BAL and sputum analysis was 63%. TBLB, when combined with BAL, did not increase diagnostic yield. Bronchoscopic findings resulted in management changes in 51% of patients. The 28-day mortality rate was 26% and was highest in patients who required mechanical ventilatory assistance before bronchoscopy.

References

1. Nguyen MH, Leather H, Clancy CJ, Cline C, Jantz MA, Kulkarni V, Wheat LJ, Wingard JR. Galactomannan testing in bronchoalveolar lavage fluid facilitates the diagnosis of invasive pulmonary aspergillosis in patients with hematologic malignancies and stem cell transplant recipients. Biol Blood Marrow Transplant 2011; 17(7): 1043-50.
2. Peikert T, Rana S, Edell ES. Safety, diagnostic yield, and therapeutic implications of flexible bronchoscopy in patients with febrile neutropenia and pulmonary infiltrates. Mayo Clin Proc 2005; 80(11): 1414-20.

Question III.2: A 52-year-old patient with non-Hodgkin lymphoma has acute respiratory failure after the second course of chemotherapy. Chest radiograph prior to intubation shows bilateral and diffuse alveolar infiltrates. Once intubated, the patient requires invasive mechanical ventilation on FiO_2 of 0.7 and PEEP of 15 cm H_2O. What should be done next?

A.   Bronchoscopy with bronchioloalveolar lavage (BAL) cytology, bacterial, viral and fungal cultures and galactomannan (GM) antigen

B.   Bronchoscopy with transbronchial lung biopsy (TBLB) and brushings for bacterial, viral and fungal cultures

C.   No bronchoscopy: start broad-spectrum antibiotics and antifungal covering aspergillosis and Mucormycosis

D.   No Bronchoscopy: perform imaging studies and microbiological studies of blood, urine, sputum, and nasopharyngeal aspirates. Begin appropriate anti-infectious therapy as soon as possible

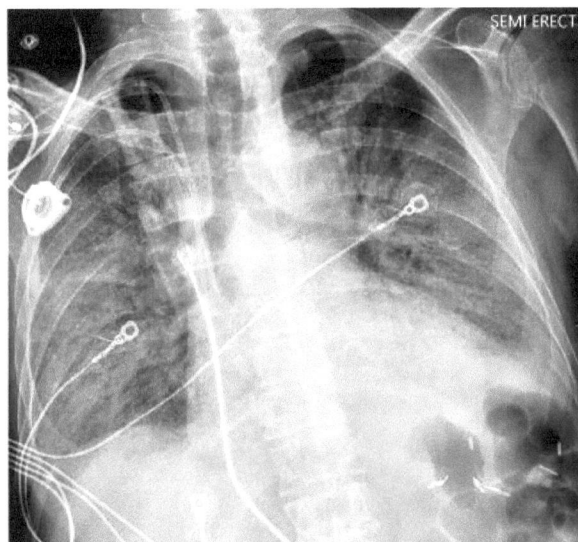

Answer III.2:   D

Diagnostic flexible bronchoscopy with BAL may prompt acute respiratory failure (ARF) and clinical deterioration in hematology and oncology patients. A diagnostic strategy that does not include bronchoscopy can indeed be as effective as bronchoscopy.

Studies show that ARF may occur in 10% to 50% of the patients with solid tumors or hematologic malignancies during the course of their illness. One prospective multi-center study of oncologic patients with ARF evaluated the diagnostic yields of noninvasive test strategies (microbiological studies of blood, urine, sputum, and nasopharyngeal aspirates) with and without bronchoscopy and BAL (1). Overall, noninvasive diagnostic tests had a diagnostic yield of 66.7% and BAL of 50.5%. BAL, however, was the only investigation that provided a diagnosis in 33.7% of the patients. Mortality was not significantly different between the groups with and without BAL; or within the BAL group, between the patients with and without a diagnosis.

In another multicenter randomized controlled trial, noninvasive testing alone was compared with noninvasive testing plus BAL in patients suffering from cancer who were not receiving ventilatory support at intensive care unit admission (2). The need for subsequent mechanical ventilation was not significantly greater in the BAL group than in the noninvasive group (35.4 vs. 38.7%; P = 0.62). The proportion of patients with no diagnosis was not smaller in the noninvasive group (21.7 vs. 20.4%; difference, -1.3% [-10.4 to 7.7]). BAL performed in the ICU did not significantly increase intubation requirements in critically ill cancer patients with ARF. In this study, noninvasive testing alone was not inferior to noninvasive testing plus BAL for identifying the cause of ARF.

Based on the results from these studies, in hypoxemic oncologic patients with ARF, a noninvasive strategy may provide a diagnosis in a significant number of cases and bronchoscopy should not be the first test in this high-risk population. BAL may have an important role in the diagnostic work-up of selected critically ill cancer patients, but should be performed only after diligent analysis of its risks and benefits and after a thorough non-invasive strategy is performed.

References

1. Azoulay E, Mokart D, Rabbat A, Pene F, Kouatchet A, Bruneel F, Vincent F, Hamidfar R, Moreau D, Mohammedi I, Epinette G, Beduneau G, Castelain V, de Lassence A, Gruson D, Lemiale V, Renard B, Chevret S, Schlemmer B. Diagnostic bronchoscopy in hematology and oncology patients with acute respiratory failure: prospective multicenter data. Crit Care Med 2008; 36(1): 100-7.
2. Azoulay E, Mokart D, Lambert J, Lemiale V, Rabbat A, Kouatchet A, Vincent F, Gruson D, Bruneel F, Epinette-Branche G, Lafabrie A, Hamidfar-Roy R, Cracco C, Renard B, Tonnelier JM, Blot F, Chevret S, Schlemmer B. Diagnostic strategy for hematology and oncology patients with acute respiratory failure: randomized controlled trial. Am J Respir Crit Care Med 2010; 182(8): 1038-46.

Question III.3: An immunocompromised patient with neutropenia and pneumonia is admitted to the intensive care unit with the chest radiograph below. Bronchoalveolar lavage (BAL) should be <u>routinely</u> performed in such patients because it impacts the choice of antimicrobial treatment in the <u>majority</u> of patients. This statement is:

A.   True
B.   False

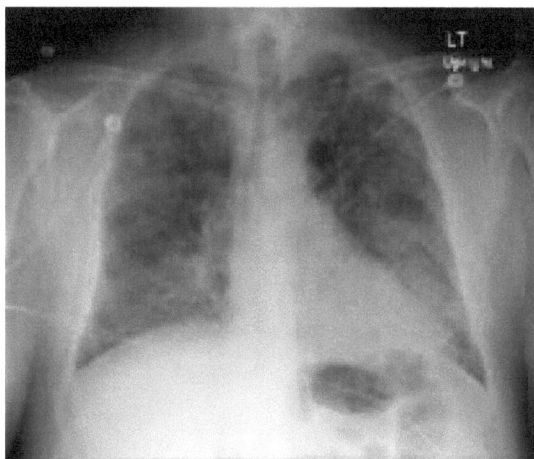

Answer III.3:   B

     One study evaluated retrospectively the impact of diagnostic bronchoscopy with BAL on treatment and outcome of pneumonia in patients with and without neutropenia (1). BAL revealed positive bacterial results in 67% of cases. There was no statistically significant difference between neutropenic (57%) and non-neutropenic (79%) patients (p = 0.076). Positive fungal cultures were found in 59% of cases. Similarly, there was no significant difference between neutropenic and non-neutropenic patients (p = 0.9). BAL results directed a change of therapy in 11% of patients (7% neutropenic and 14% non-neutropenic). Overall mortality related to pneumonia was 16% in this study. There was no significant difference in mortality between neutropenic and non-neutropenic patients (p = 0.8). There was also no difference in mortality rate for cases with positive or negative BAL results (p = 0.3). In this patient population, the yield of BAL rarely had a significant influence on treatment and outcome of pneumonia. The authors thus concluded that BAL had a low impact on the choice of antimicrobial treatment.

     More pertinent to ICU physicians, a prospective study evaluated the impact of bronchoscopy and BAL on guiding the treatment and ICU clinical outcome in neutropenic patients with pulmonary infiltrates (2). The patients were classified into two groups according to the cause of neutropenia (due to high-dose chemotherapy or stem cell transplantation (SCT). BAL in this neutropenic population had an acceptable overall diagnostic yield (49%), with a significantly better yield in the ICU patients with high-dose chemotherapy-induced neutropenia (63%). Patients who had a diagnostic BAL that changed therapy did not survive longer than patients who had a BAL that did not change therapy. The authors concluded that the use of routine diagnostic BAL in ICU neutropenic patients with pulmonary infiltrates was difficult to establish, even if BAL was helpful in the management of these critically ill patients. Although BAL had a low complication rate, it infrequently led to a change in treatment and was not associated with improved patient survival in the ICU.

References

1. Kuehnhardt D, Hannemann M, Schmidt B, Heider U, Possinger K, Eucker J. Therapeutic implication of BAL in patients with neutropenia. Ann Hematol 2009; 88(12): 1249-56.
2. Gruson D, Hilbert G, Valentino R, Vargas F, Chene G, Bebear C, Allery A, Pigneux A, Gbikpi-Benissan G, Cardinaud JP. Utility of fiberoptic bronchoscopy in neutropenic patients admitted to the intensive care unit with pulmonary infiltrates. Crit Care Med 2000; 28(7): 2224-30.

Question III.4: In a patient with acute respiratory distress syndrome (ARDS) and suspected pulmonary Blastomycosis based on epidemiologic data, bronchoscopic bronchial washings have a higher diagnostic yield than bronchoscopic lung biopsy (BLB):

A. True
B. False

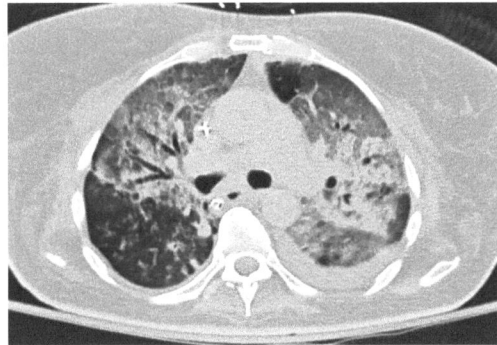

Answer III.4: A

Blastomycosis is an endemic mycosis that occurs predominantly in North America and mostly involves the lungs. Definitive diagnosis is made by isolation of *B. dermatitidis* in culture. In patients with pulmonary Blastomycosis, diagnostic yield is high for both bronchoscopy and sputum samples (1). Direct visualization of *B. dermatitidis* in fluid or tissues can lead to a rapid presumptive diagnosis of Blastomycosis and initiation of antifungal therapy.

Blastomycosis is associated with a spectrum of illness ranging from subclinical infection to acute or chronic pneumonia; a subset of individuals with acute pulmonary Blastomycosis can progress to fulminant multilobar pneumonia and ARDS (2). Diffuse pulmonary infiltrates associated with ARDS occur infrequently but are associated with a high mortality rate. Pulmonary Blastomycosis often mimics bacterial pneumonia which may result in delayed antifungal therapy or performance of unnecessary diagnostic procedures. *B. dermatitidis* can be isolated from respiratory secretions in most patients with a lung infection. In one study, bronchoscopy was diagnostic in 92% of patients (3). Cultures of specimens from bronchial washings and BAL were positive in 100% and 67% of cases, respectively. The results of testing pathologic specimens from BLB, bronchial brushings, and bronchoscopic needle aspiration were positive in 22%, 50%, and 0% of specimens, respectively. These data suggest that sputum samples and bronchial washings should be the initial tests in patients with suspected Blastomycosis.

References

1. Castillo CG, Kauffman CA, Miceli MH. Blastomycosis. Infect Dis Clin North Am 2015 pii: S0891-5520(15)00091-4.
2. Chapman SW, Dismukes WE, Proia LA, Bradsher RW, Pappas PG, Threlkeld MG, Kauffman CA; Infectious Diseases Society of America. Clinical practice guidelines for the management of Blastomycosis: 2008 update by the Infectious Diseases Society of America. Clin Infect Dis 2008; 46(12): 1801-12.
3. Martynowicz MA, Prakash UB. Pulmonary Blastomycosis: an appraisal of diagnostic techniques. Chest 2002; 121(3): 768-73.

Question III.5: A 67-year-old immunocompetent patient develops fever and a new right lower lobe infiltrate four days after being intubated for following traumatic chest injury and intracerebral bleeding. A diagnosis of ventilator-associated pneumonia (VAP) is suspected. Which of the following strategies should be used?

A.   Bronchoscopy with brushings and BAL quantitative cultures
B.   Endotracheal aspirate non-quantitative analysis
C.   Bronchoscopy with transbronchial lung biopsy

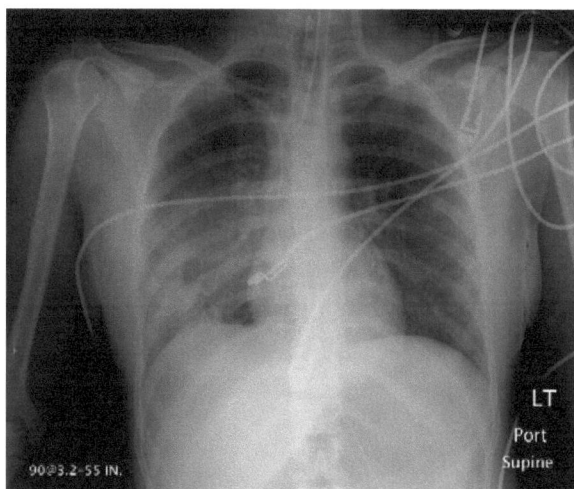

Answer III.5:   B

Several original studies and systematic reviews evaluated the effect on clinical outcome and antibiotic use of two VAP diagnostic strategies including invasive and noninvasive (1, 2, 3). The invasive management strategy is comprised of bronchoscopic protected specimen brush samples or bronchoalveolar lavage samples and their quantitative cultures. The noninvasive ("clinical") management strategy is based on clinical criteria and potential isolation of microorganisms by non-quantitative analysis of endotracheal aspirates.

In a meta-analysis, (3), authors report results from four randomized trials comparing lower respiratory tract sampling and quantitative culture with clinical criteria for the diagnosis of ventilator-associated pneumonia. They note that the likelihood of modifying initial antimicrobial therapy in the sampling group was almost three times that in the clinical-criteria group. They also state that in patient populations with a low prevalence of infection or colonization with antibiotic-resistant bacteria, the use of endotracheal aspiration should suffice, because initial empirical treatment with broad-spectrum antimicrobial agents is not required. In addition to emphasizing the importance of appropriate antibiotic selection, they insist on the clinician's responsibility to diminish risks of subsequent antibiotic resistance by using a strategy of de-escalation (appropriate narrow and selective treatment of short duration).

Another landmark randomized controlled study compared the two strategies (4). Patients who received invasive management had reduced mortality at day 14 (16.2% and 25.8%; P = 0.022), decreased mean Sepsis-related Organ Failure Assessment scores at day 3 (6.1+/-4.0 and 7.0+/-4.3; P = 0.033) and day 7 (4.9+/-4.0 and 5.8+/-4.4; P = 0.043), and decreased antibiotic use (mean number of antibiotic-free days, 5.0+/-5.1 and 2.2+/-3.5; P < 0.001). At 28 days, the invasive management group had significantly more antibiotic-free days (11.5+/-9.0 compared with 7.5+/-7.6; P < 0.001), and only multivariate analysis showed a significant difference in mortality (hazard ratio, 1.54 [CI, 1.10 to 2.16]; P = 0.01). Compared with a noninvasive management strategy, an invasive management strategy was associated with significantly fewer deaths at 14 days, earlier attenuation of organ dysfunction, and less antibiotic use in patients suspected of having ventilator-associated pneumonia.

This strategy increases the likelihood that true pathogens are identified while minimizing unnecessary antimicrobial therapy. Subsequent studies, however, showed that two diagnostic strategies for VAP (BAL with quantitative culture of the fluid and endotracheal aspiration with nonquantitative culture of the aspirate) are associated with similar clinical outcomes and similar use of antimicrobials (3).

References

1. Shorr AF, Sherner JH, Jackson WL, Kollef MH. Invasive approaches to the diagnosis of ventilator-associated pneumonia: a meta-analysis. Crit Care Med 2005; 33(1): 46-53.
2. Berton DC, Kalil AC, Teixeira PJ. Quantitative versus qualitative cultures of respiratory secretions for clinical outcomes in patients with ventilator-associated pneumonia. Cochrane Database Syst Rev 2014; 10: CD006482.
3. Canadian Critical Care Trials Group. A randomized trial of diagnostic techniques for ventilator-associated pneumonia. N Engl J Med 2006; 355(25): 2619-30.
4. Fagon JY, Chastre J, Wolff M, Gervais C, Parer-Aubas S, Stéphan F, Similowski T, Mercat A, Diehl JL, Sollet JP, Tenaillon A. Invasive and noninvasive strategies for management of suspected ventilator-associated pneumonia. A randomized trial. Ann Intern Med 2000; 132(8): 621-30.

Question III.6: In addition to diagnosing possible stenosis, there are multiple indications for bronchoscopy in lung transplant patients. Which of the following statements is <u>correct</u> regarding bronchoscopy in transplant recipients admitted to the Intensive Care Unit?

A. Transbronchial lung biopsy should be avoided in transplant recipients because of the increased risk of pneumothorax.

B. Bronchoscopy assists in the evaluation and diagnosis of primary graft dysfunction including infection and rejection.

C. Clinically indicated bronchoscopy has been repeatedly shown to be of greater benefit for diagnosing lung rejection than routinely scheduled surveillance bronchoscopy in lung transplant recipients.

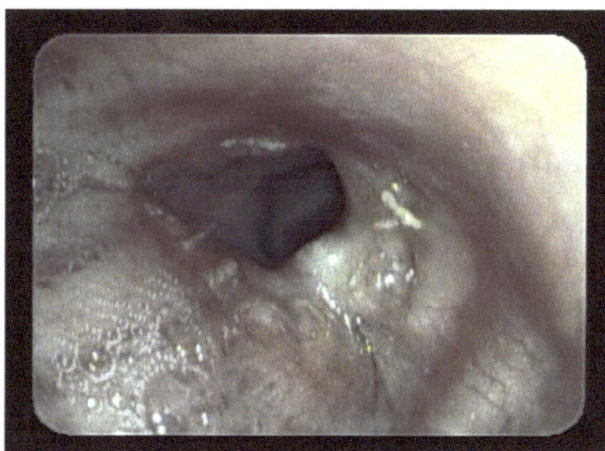

Left main bronchial stenosis after
lung transplantation

Answer III.6:   B

There are concerns about bronchoscopy safety in critically ill transplant patients because it may cause hemorrhage, pneumothorax, prolonged hypoxemia and pneumonia. However, bronchoscopy does add value in this population and can change management in a significant proportion of patients.

Lung transplant patients may be admitted to the ICU for primary graft dysfunction (PGD), pulmonary infections due to immunosuppression or for other complications related to the surgery. The prevention and early detection of post-transplantation rejection and infection are relevant to achieving long-term survival after lung transplantation. Bronchoscopy may be useful in these patients because these complications can be potentially detected using bronchoscopy with inspection, bronchoalveolar lavage (BAL), and transbronchial lung biopsy (TBLB).

Surveillance bronchoscopy post-transplant (SB) is performed in many centers. In these regards, the clinical utility of SB after lung transplantation was evaluated by comparing it with clinically indicated bronchoscopy (CIB) in one retrospective study (1). There was no significant difference in TBLB/BAL-positivity and intervention rates between the SBs and CIBs. As to complications associated with SB, moderate hemorrhage was observed in 11% of the patients, and pneumothorax was found in 1% of the patients. No patients required transfusion. One patient underwent surgery for prolonged air leak after SB. The authors concluded that SB detected rejection and airway infection or colonization with minimum complications, especially within 12 months after lung transplantation.

In another retrospective study with a cohort of 76 lung transplant recipients who underwent bronchoscopy and were admitted to medical intensive care unit (MICU), bronchoscopy was helpful for the evaluation and management of airway complications [secretion clearance (18% bronchoscopy procedures), stenosis/dehiscence (8% patients)] and for optimizing the management of lower respiratory tract infections. Isolation of resistant gram-negative organisms, community-acquired respiratory viruses, and fungi commonly led to modification in antimicrobial therapy in 35% of cases (2). A nonspecific finding of acute lung injury was seen on histopathology evaluation in 70% of patients who underwent transbronchial biopsy. Hypoxia (3%) and hypotension (3%), but no mortality was reported in this series.

References

1. Inoue M, Minami M, Wada N, Nakagiri T, Funaki S, Kawamura T, Shintani Y, Okumura M. Results of surveillance bronchoscopy after cadaveric lung transplantation: a Japanese single-institution study. Transplant Proc 2014; 46(3): 944-7.
2. Mohanka MR, Mehta AC, Budev MM, Machuzak MS, Gildea TR. Impact of bedside bronchoscopy in critically ill lung transplant recipients. J Bronchology Interv Pulmonol 2014; 21(3): 199-207.

Question III.7: Bronchoalveolar lavage should be routinely performed in patients with acute myeloid leukemia (AML) admitted to intensive care unit for acute respiratory failure.

A.   Yes
B.   No

Answer III.7:   B

In one study addressing this question, BAL was performed in 121 patients with hematologic malignancy admitted to ICU (1). The authors reported life-threatening complications in 10% of patients. The overall diagnostic yield of BAL was 47% in AML patients and 50% in Lymphoid Malignancy (LM) including non–Hodgkin's lymphoma, Hodgkin's lymphoma, chronic lymphoid leukemia and multiple myeloma patients. A microorganism was isolated from BAL in 23% of AML patients and 41% of LM patients (P<0.005). BAL resulted in significant therapeutic changes in 17% of AML patients vs. 35% of LM patients (P=0.039). This study suggests a low diagnostic yield of BAL for infections and the low rate of therapeutic changes in unselected AML patients with ARF admitted in ICU. In contrast, BAL was found to be more helpful in patients with Lymphoid Malignancy (LM).

Another study retrospectively evaluated the feasibility and the diagnostic significance of BAL samples from febrile patients with hematologic malignancies including acute leukemia (n=103), malignant lymphoma (n=84), and other malignancies or chronic neutropenia (n=12) and pulmonary infiltrates during and outside episodes of neutropenia (2); 30% of the BAL samples showed no infectious organisms; 22% showed findings classified as contamination or colonization, but 48% showed positive microbiological results including bacteria and/or fungi classified as true pathogens. Three nonlethal complications (bleeding, arrhythmia) occurred that prompted early termination of bronchoscopy. In 38.2% of patients, antibiotic treatment was modified as a result of microbiological findings from BAL samples. Thus, this study showed that BAL is a valuable diagnostic tool with a relatively low complication rates in febrile patients with hematologic malignancies and pulmonary infiltrates.

References

1. Rabbat A, Chaoui D, Lefebvre A, Roche N, Legrand O, Lorut C, Rio B, Marie JP, Huchon G. Is BAL useful in patients with acute myeloid leukemia admitted in ICU for severe respiratory complications? Leukemia 2008; 22(7): 1361-7.
2. Hummel M, Rudert S, Hof H, Hehlmann R, Buchheidt D. Diagnostic yield of bronchoscopy with bronchoalveolar lavage in febrile patients with hematologic malignancies and pulmonary infiltrates. Ann Hematol 2008; 87(4): 291-7.

Question III.8: Routine diagnostic bronchoscopy is least useful in the critically ill patient admitted to the ICU for:

A.   Pneumonia
B.   Hemoptysis
C.   Thoracic trauma
D.   Atelectasis

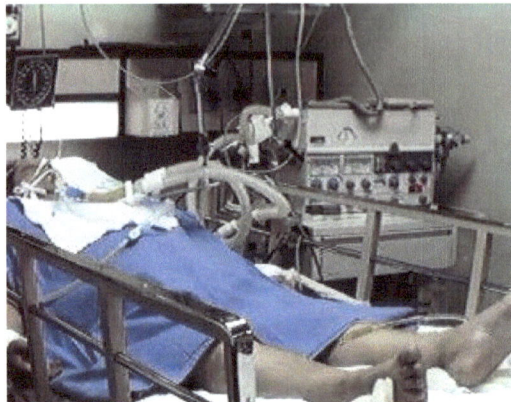

Answer III.8:   D

The indications of bronchoscopy in the ICU can be classified into diagnostic and therapeutic (1). Primary diagnostic indications include pneumonia, hemoptysis, thoracic trauma (for possible tracheal or bronchial injury), airway obstruction, inhalation injury and vocal cord function assessment.

There are obvious circumstances in which the airway examination serves multiple purposes. These include hemoptysis in a patient with bronchial obstruction caused by an aspirated foreign object or endobronchial tumor; in such cases, a therapeutic intervention can be offered as part of the procedure.

Other major therapeutic indications for performing bronchoscopy in critically ill patients include endotracheal intubation, atelectasis (resulting in gas exchange abnormalities and refractory to pulmonary hygiene measures), tracheobronchial obstruction, foreign body removal, hemoptysis, and to guide percutaneous tracheostomy.

In general, absolute contraindications of bronchoscopy include 1) noncooperation or refusal by the patient; 2) an inexperienced bronchoscopist, lack of suitable facilities or equipment; and 3) inability to maintain adequate oxygenation during the procedure ($SpO_2 < 90\%$ despite oxygen supplementation) (2). All patients should be monitored by continuous pulse oximetry during bronchoscopy. Oxygen supplementation should be routinely used and F_iO_2 or flow increased when desaturation is significant ($SpO_2 > 4\%$ change, or $SpO_2 < 90\%$) and prolonged (>1 min) to reduce the risk of hypoxemia-related complications.

Regardless of the indications or circumstances for bronchoscopy in the intensive care unit, informed consent should be obtained from the patient and/or family members. Ideally, informed consent is obtained by the physicians performing the procedure. Risks and benefits, alternatives to performing the procedure, including consequences of not performing the procedure should be covered in a way that is understandable by the patient and family members.

References

1. Guerreiro da Cunha Fragoso E, Gonçalves JM. Role of fiberoptic bronchoscopy in intensive care unit: current practice. J Bronchology Interv Pulmonol 2011; 18(1): 69-83.
2. Du Rand IA, Blaikley J, Booton R, Chaudhuri N, Gupta V, Khalid S, Mandal S, Martin J, Mills J, Navani N, Rahman NM, Wrightson JM, Munavvar M; British Thoracic Society Bronchoscopy Guideline Group. British Thoracic Society guideline for diagnostic flexible bronchoscopy in adults: accredited by NICE. Thorax 2013; 68 Suppl 1:i1-i44.
3. Informed Consent synopsis (Free download), https://www.bronchoscopy.org/wp-content/uploads/INFORMED-CONSENT-SYNOPSIS.pdf

Question III.9: A 70-year-old male patient suffering from Alzheimer's disease was admitted to the intensive care unit (ICU) with a diagnosis of aspiration pneumonia after being emergently intubated. He immediately developed fever and hypoxemia. A new infiltrate was noted in the right lower lobe on postintubation chest radiography. Early bronchoscopy could improve the outcome of this patient:

A.   True
B.   False

Answer III.9:   A

Diagnostic bronchoscopy with bronchoalveolar lavage (BAL) could be helpful for patients with aspiration-induced lung injury in order to potentially reveal causative organisms and subsequently determine the appropriate duration of antibiotic treatment. Initial administration of appropriate antibiotics can lower the mortality rate in these patients.

A retrospective cohort study analyzed the role of bronchoscopy in patients with aspiration who were mechanically ventilated in a medical ICU (1). Patients were divided into early bronchoscopy (EB) (bronchoscopy ≤24 h after intubation) and late bronchoscopy (LB) (bronchoscopy >24 h after intubation) groups. The EB showed significantly lower in-ICU and 90-day mortality (in-ICU: 4.9% vs 24.6%; 90-day: 11.8 vs 32.8%) regardless of the initial empirical antibiotics. In addition, their sequential organ failure assessment score on day 7 tended to decrease more rapidly. Among the survivors, patients in the EB group were extubated earlier with a higher success rate, had a shorter length of mechanical ventilation and had a shorter ICU stay. The early bronchoscopy was associated with lower 90-day mortality in multivariate analysis (odds ratio: 0.412; 95% confidence interval: 0.192–0.883). In addition to performing diagnostic BAL, early bronchoscopy could benefit mechanically ventilated patients with aspiration pneumonia by suctioning of aspirated foreign material.

References

1. Lee HW, Min J, Park J, Lee YJ, Kim SJ, Park JS, Yoon HI, Lee JH, Lee CT, Cho YJ. Clinical impact of early bronchoscopy in mechanically ventilated patients with aspiration pneumonia. Respirology 2015; 20(7): 1115-22.

Question III.10: A 30-year-old female was admitted to the intensive care unit (ICU) with hypoxemia and was promptly intubated and placed on mechanical ventilation. Bilateral diffuse opacities were noted on chest radiography (see Figure). The patient's relatives told the ICU team that she had a fever and pleuritic chest pain for one week prior to admission. Bronchoscopy with bronchoalveolar lavage (BAL) was performed. BAL eosinophilia (> 25%) was detected on the differential WBC count. Which of the following diseases is the most probable diagnosis in this patient?

A.   Acute interstitial pneumonia
B.   Hypersensitivity pneumonitis
C.   Acute eosinophilic pneumonia
D.   Acute respiratory distress syndrome

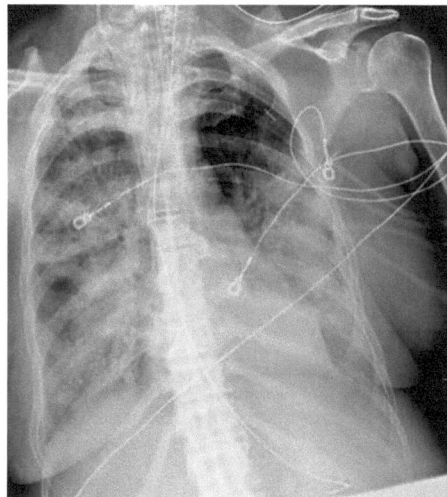

Answer III.10:   C

　　Acute eosinophilic pneumonia (AEP) is a severe and rapidly progressive lung disease that can cause respiratory failure (1). AEP can mimic other diseases causing acute respiratory distress syndrome or severe community-acquired pneumonia, so the diagnosis could be delayed. The cause of this disease in the majority of patients is unknown, even though some cases may be caused by smoke inhalation, inhaled dust or drugs.

　　Patients with AEP present with rapid onset of cough, tachypnea, and dyspnea in otherwise previously healthy individuals. Symptoms progress from mild dyspnea to life-threatening respiratory failure in only a few hours. Fever is usually present over 38 degrees Celsius. Pleuritic chest pain and myalgias are common symptoms. Diagnosis is established by bronchoalveolar lavage. AEP shows increased eosinophils in BAL fluid of an average percentage of 37% to 54% eosinophils on differential cell count, with sterile bacterial cultures. Chest X-ray shows a pattern consistent with pulmonary edema, with extensive airspace opacities, interlobular septal thickening, and even pleural effusions. The infiltrates are diffuse and not peripherally based, as in chronic eosinophilic pneumonia. Patients with Acute Eosinophilic Pneumonia have a rapid and very good response to corticosteroids. Contrary to chronic eosinophilic pneumonia, a relatively short course of steroids of 2 weeks is usually enough, and rebound after discontinuation of treatment (as seen in chronic disease) does not occur.

References

1. Sohn JW. Acute eosinophilic pneumonia. Tuberc Respir Dis (Seoul) 2013; 74(2): 51-5.

Question III.11: A 68-year-old man (body weight 75 kg) was hospitalized for dyspnea and a right lower lobe (RLL) infiltrate not responding to two courses of broad-spectrum antibiotics. Patient had no previous cardiac, pulmonary, liver or neurologic conditions. PET CT scan was performed for suspected malignancy and it showed intense fluorodeoxyglucose (FDG) uptake in the RLL infiltrate but no other abnormalities. Flexible bronchoscopy was performed under moderate sedation with a total of 2 mg of midazolam, 25 micrograms of fentanyl and 200 mg of 1% lidocaine. Transbronchial lung biopsy (TBLB) was performed from the lateral segment of the RLL. Immediately following the biopsy, the patient had a seizure and became unresponsive with signs of upper airways obstruction requiring administration of high flow oxygen. Which of the following is the most likely explanation for this patient's symptoms?

A. Lidocaine overdose resulting in seizure
B. Cerebral air embolism following TBLB
C. Over sedation and hypercarbic encephalopathy

Answer III.11: B

Cerebral air embolism following TBLB and even transbronchial needle aspiration (TBNA) is a very rare but potentially fatal complication. The bronchoscopist should be aware of this rare complication, especially in patients, becoming unresponsive with acute neurologic signs during or immediately following bronchoscopy (1).

Two mechanisms are necessary for air embolism to occur: 1) a site of air entry resulting from a defect in a vessel wall from the biopsy and 2) a pressure gradient which forces the air bubbles through the defect (2). The abnormal surrounding lung tissue caused by the underlying disease process (i.e. tumor, pneumonia) may prevent the normally protective vasoconstriction that helps occlude these defects. Cerebral air emboli can lead to decreased or loss of consciousness, focal neurological deficits and seizures.

The diagnosis of air embolism is based on symptoms that occur after a potential precipitating event. Demonstration of intra-vascular bubbles can be difficult (as they are transient). CT scan may occasionally show minute air bubbles in cerebral vessels and brain MRI will show signs of acute ischemia. The management of suspected air embolism consists of emergent Trendelenburg position, adding high-flow oxygen, discontinuing nitrous oxide if used for anesthesia, and supportive measures including avoidance of positive pressure ventilation (this may increase the pressure gradient thereby increasing the volume of embolized air) and hyperbaric oxygen.

Lidocaine toxicity is unlikely in this patient given the minimal dose used (200 mg). Cardiac, gastrointestinal and neurologic toxicity can occur seen when the maximum dose is exceeded (~ 7 mg/kg) or in patients with impaired metabolism (cardiac or liver disease). over sedation is unlikely given the minimal dose of midazolam and fentanyl.

References

1. Azzola A, von Garnier C, Chhajed PN, Schirp U, Tamm M. Fatal cerebral air embolism following uneventful flexible bronchoscopy. Respiration 2010; 80(6): 569-72.
2. Evison M, Crosbie PA, Bright-Thomas R, Alaloul M, Booton R. Cerebral air embolism following transbronchial lung biopsy during flexible bronchoscopy. Respir Med Case Rep 2014; 12: 39-40.

Question III.12: Which one of the following drugs can be continued prior to performing transbronchial lung biopsy (TBLB)?

A.   Clopidogrel
B.   Ticlodipine
C.   Prasugrel
D.   Aspirin

Answer III.12:   D

Clopidogrel (Plavix), ticlopidine (Ticlid) and prasugrel (Effient) should be stopped for 5-7 days before TBLB (1, 2, 3). Aspirin alone can be continued. As with any procedure, the risks of biopsy need to be weighed against the potential benefits and a meaningful informed consent should be obtained from patient and or family. It is thus relevant to carefully review patient's medication list (current and prior to ICU admission) prior to performing a bronchoscopic lung biopsy. Airway bleeding in critically ill patients may be poorly tolerated given the prevalence of impaired gas exchange encountered in these patients.

References

1. Jain P, Hadique S, Mehta AC. Transbronchial lung biopsy. A.C. Mehta and P. Jain (eds.), Interventional Bronchoscopy: A Clinical Guide, Respiratory Medicine 10, DOI 10. 1007/978-1-62703-395-4_2, Springer Science+Business Media New York 2010.
2. Ernst A, Eberhardt R, Wahidi M, Becker HD, Herth FJ. Effect of routine clopidogrel use on bleeding complications after transbronchial biopsy in humans. Chest. 2006;129(3):734-7.
3. Todd H. Baron, M.D., Patrick S. Kamath, M.D., and Robert D. McBane, M.D. Management of Antithrombotic Therapy in Patients Undergoing Invasive Procedures. N Engl J Med 2013; 368:2113-2124.

Question III.13: Studies <u>consistently</u> show that bronchoscopic grading of the degree of airway inhalation injury predicts mortality in burn patients admitted to the ICU. This statement is:

A.   True
B.   False

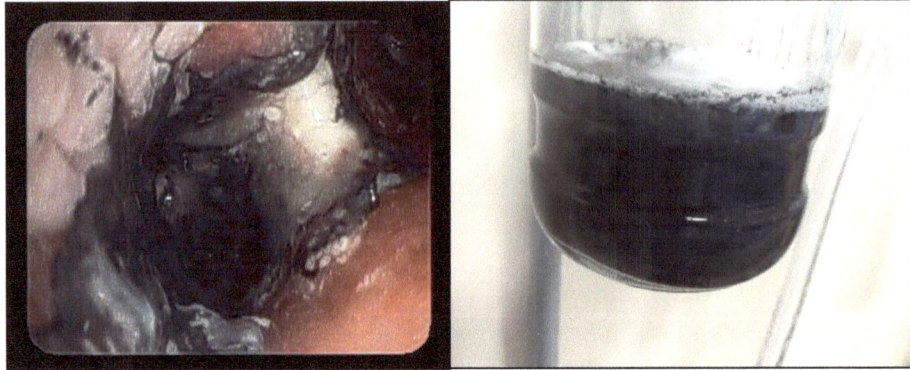

Answer III.13:   B

Inhalation injury is a risk factor for increased morbidity and mortality and its incidence is approximately 10–20% among burn patients. Inhalation injury assessment based on clinical evaluation is subjective and does not indicate the severity of the injury. Diagnosis and severity can be confirmed by bronchoscopy within 24 h of the burn. In a prospective, observational study consisted of 192 burn patients who underwent bronchoscopy within 24 h, however, there was no difference between upper airway and lower airway inhalation injury confirmed by bronchoscopy (1). In this study, bronchoscopic severity grades and mechanical ventilation but not arterial O_2 pressure $(PaO_2)/FiO_2$ predicted the mortality of burn patients with inhalation injury.

However, a retrospective review of all patients requiring more than 48 hours of mechanical ventilation investigated whether the severity of the mucosal injury predicts clinically meaningful outcomes (2). This study showed conflicting results. Bronchoscopy was performed on all subjects at admission and grading of severity was documented using the grades 0 to 4 abbreviated injury score (AIS). Subjects with grade 1 or 2 injury were considered the low-grade group, whereas those with grade 3 or 4 injury, the high-grade group. Subjects with high-grade injury showed statistically insignificant trends toward larger 48-hour fluid volumes (P = 0.07), poorer oxygenation over the first 3 post-burn days (P = 0.055), longer duration of ventilation (P = 0.08), and fewer ventilator-free days (P = 0.047) compared with the low-grade group. High-grade and low-grade injury groups did not differ significantly in the incidence of acute respiratory distress syndrome or mortality. The individual grades of the 0 to

4 severity grading scale were not relevant in predicting outcomes in this population of adult burn patients.

References

1. You K, Yang HT, Kym D, Yoon J, Haejun Yim, Cho YS, Hur J, Chun W, Kim JH. Inhalation injury in burn patients: establishing the link between diagnosis and prognosis. Burns 2014; 40(8): 1470-5.
2. Spano S, Hanna S, Li Z, Wood D, Cartotto R. Does Bronchoscopic Evaluation of Inhalation Injury Severity Predict Outcome? J Burn Care Res 2016; 37(1): 1-11.

Question III.14: A 44-year- old woman presents with dyspnea and severe hypoxemia requiring F_iO_2 of 1 via non-rebreather face mask. Shortly after admission to the ICU, the patient decompensated and required endotracheal intubation and invasive mechanical ventilation (Assist Control with Tidal Volume 400 ml; Respiratory Rate 20, PEEP 12, FIO2 0.7). Bilateral diffuse ground-glass opacities were noted on chest radiography and computed tomography (see figure below). Bronchoscopy with bronchoalveolar lavage (BAL) showed abundant hemosiderin-laden macrophages in the lavage fluid from the right upper lobe anterior segment and right middle lobe lateral segment. Which of the following is the most probable diagnosis in this patient?

A.   Diffuse alveolar hemorrhage
B.   Acute respiratory distress syndrome
C.   Acute cryptogenic pneumonia

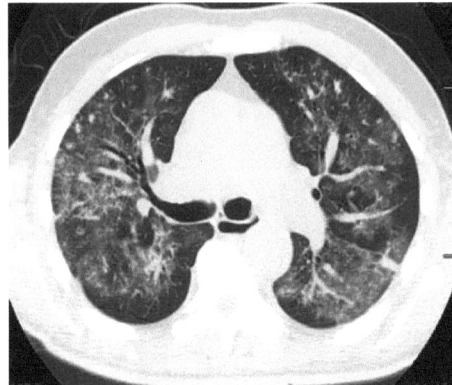

Answer III.14:   A

Diffuse alveolar hemorrhage (DAH) is a life-threatening syndrome caused by a variety of disorders associated with hemoptysis, anemia, diffuse lung infiltrates, and acute respiratory failure (1); about a third of patients with DAH do not have hemoptysis. Early bronchoscopy is indicated in most patients who are suspected to have DAH as bronchoscopic findings are diagnostic and help exclude infectious etiologies. BAL iron staining revealing more than 20% hemosiderin-laden macrophages (HLM) among all alveolar macrophages support for a diagnosis of DAH (2). The presence of HLM is not restricted to DAH, however, and is also commonly seen in patients with diffuse alveolar damage (as seen in ARDS). A progressively bloodier return during the BAL maneuver also supports the diagnosis of DAH.

ARDS usually has an obvious trigger such as infection, trauma, pancreatitis or aspiration of gastric content. Acute cryptogenic organizing pneumonia can present in a similar fashion, but the BAL cell count differential shows neutrophilia and the infiltrates tend to be patchier in distribution.

Management of DAH involves supportive care including ventilatory support ranging from oxygen supplementation to mechanical ventilation (2,3). The coagulation cascade should be evaluated, and coagulation abnormalities should be corrected accordingly. Commonly accepted targets include a platelet count > 50,000/µl and an INR < 1.5. It is crucial to identify and treat the underlying etiology of the DAH. Non-immune etiologies are treated by addressing the cause e.g. heart failure management or discontinuation of any causative drugs. High-dose methylprednisolone therapy is critical to quickly control the inflammatory activity in immune-mediated DAH (e.g. Churg Strauss disease, Granulomatosis with polyangiitis, Goodpasture syndrome). Glucocorticoids are frequently started while diagnostic test results are pending. Most noteworthy is that among three possible causes of DAH: (1) DAD, (2) bland pulmonary hemorrhage and (3) capillaritis (immune-mediated or not), only the latter is best treated with corticosteroids.

References

1. Park MS. Diffuse alveolar hemorrhage. Tuberc Respir Dis (Seoul) 2013; 74(4): 151-62.
2. Krause ML, Cartin-Ceba R, Specks U, Peikert T. Update on diffuse alveolar hemorrhage and pulmonary vasculitis. Immunol Allergy Clin North Am 2012; 32(4): 587-600.
3. Maldonado F, Parambil JG, Yi ES, Decker PA, Ryu JH. Hemosiderin-laden macrophages in the bronchoalveolar lavage fluid of patients with diffuse alveolar damage. Eur Respir J. 2009 Jun;33(6):1361-66.

Question III.15: A 75-year- old man with fever and a right lower lobe infiltrate was admitted to the Oncology ward for suspected community-acquired pneumonia. He was treated with intravenous ticarcillin/clavulanic acid and azithromycin. He had a diagnosis of HIV (last CD_4 count 150) and a new diagnosis of pancreatic cancer for which he received chemotherapy ten days prior to admission. Given persistent fever and development of neutropenia and hypoxemia, the patient was transferred to the ICU where he received oxygen supplementation with facemask of F_iO_2 0.5. High resolution computed tomography (HRCT) detected diffuse patchy ground-glass opacities (GGO) and interstitial thickening. Microscopic sputum examination was non-diagnostic and blood cultures for bacteria and fungi were negative. Viral serological testing for cytomegalovirus antigen pp65 was likewise negative. Bronchoalveolar lavage (BAL) was performed. Which one of the following is the most likely diagnosis?

A.   Pneumocystis (carinii) jiroveci pneumonia (PCP)
B.   Invasive pulmonary aspergillosis
C.   Smear-negative pulmonary tuberculosis
D.   Acute hypersensitivity pneumonitis

Answer III.15:   A

Pneumocystis (carinii) jiroveci pneumonia (PCP) usually occurs in immunocompromised individuals, especially hematopoietic stem cell and solid organ transplant recipients and those receiving immunosuppressive agents. It is the most common opportunistic infection in persons with advanced human immunodeficiency virus (HIV) infection (1). An indolent time course is characteristic in HIV-infected patients. Fulminant respiratory failure associated with fever and dry cough is more often seen in non-HIV-infected patients.

Although the microscopic demonstration of the organisms in respiratory specimens of induced sputum, bronchoalveolar lavage (BAL) fluid, or lung tissue is still the "gold standard" of diagnosing PCP (Cultures are not available). For *P jiroveci*, polymerase chain reaction has a high sensitivity (2). Serum β-D-glucan is useful as an adjunctive tool for the diagnosis of PCP. Patchy or diffuse GGO, interstitial thickening and/or air-space consolidation showed high sensitivity (86.7%) and specificity (96.8%) for PCP in populations at high risk for this infection (3). Trimethoprim–sulfamethoxazole and corticosteroids are the first-line agents for the treatment of severe PCP. Indications for steroids, although not evidence-based, include Pa02<70 and AaDO>35.

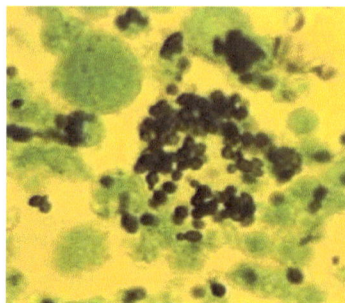

References

1. Gilroy SA, Bennett NJ. Pneumocystis pneumonia. Semin Respir Crit Care Med 2011; 32(6): 775-82.
2. Tasaka S. Pneumocystis Pneumonia in Human Immunodeficiency Virus-infected Adults and Adolescents: Current Concepts and Future Directions. Clin Med Insights Circ Respir Pulm Med 2015; 9(Suppl 1): 19-28.
3. Kang M, Deoghuria D, Varma S, Gupta D, Bhatia A, Khandelwal N. Role of HRCT in detection and characterization of pulmonary abnormalities in patients with febrile neutropenia. Lung India 2013; 30(2): 124-30.

Question III.16: Critically ill non-intubated patients with hypoxemic respiratory failure undergoing bronchoscopy in the intensive care unit have an increased risk of hypoxemia-related complications. Which one of the following should be used during the procedure to prevent bronchoscopy-related complications in this patient population?

A.   High-flow nasal cannula (HFNC)
B.   Non-invasive ventilation (NIV)
C.   Endotracheal tube (ETT)

Answer III.16:   B

Flexible bronchoscopy is frequently performed to diagnose and treat treatment patients with respiratory illness in the intensive care unit (ICU). While bronchoscopy is generally considered safe, critically ill patients undergoing bronchoscopy are at an increased risk for complications, most of which are related to worsening of pre-existing hypoxemia.

A prospective randomized trial compared HFNC and NIV in patients with acute hypoxemic respiratory failure undergoing flexible bronchoscopy. The study assessed the ability to maintain adequate oxygen saturation during bronchoscopy, changes in gas exchange and clinical outcome post-bronchoscopy (1). After the initiation of NIV and HFNC, oxygen levels were significantly higher in the NIV group compared to the HFNC group. Thus, the application of NIV is superior to HFNC in regards to oxygenation before, during and after bronchoscopy in patients with moderate to severe hypoxemia.

In addition to severe refractory hypoxemia, other indications for NIV during bronchoscopy include obstructive sleep apnea and obesity hypoventilation syndrome, bronchoscopy in pediatric patients, postoperative respiratory distress, severe chronic obstructive pulmonary disease and expiratory central-airway collapse (2). Bronchoscopy on NIV may be an alternative to endotracheal intubation in these high-risk patients.

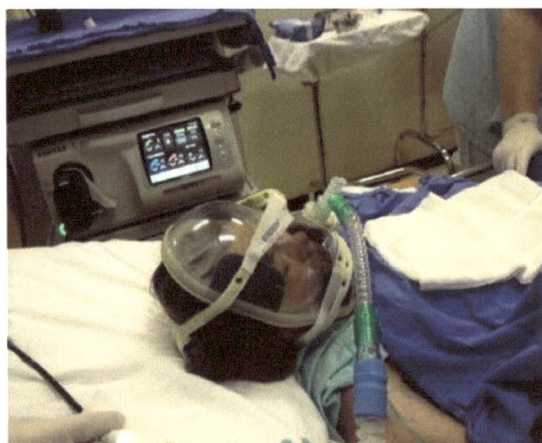

Example of full face mask
Noninvasive Positive Pressure Ventilation

References

1. Simon M, Braune S, Frings D, Wiontzek AK, Klose H, Kluge S. High-flow nasal cannula oxygen versus non-invasive ventilation in patients with acute hypoxemic respiratory failure undergoing flexible bronchoscopy--a prospective randomized trial. Crit Care 2014; 18(6): 712.
2. Murgu SD, Pecson J, Colt HG. Bronchoscopy during noninvasive ventilation: indications and technique. Respir Care 2010; 55(5): 595-600.

Question III.17: A 75-year-old female underwent a diagnostic bronchoscopy. Immediately post procedure, she develops respiratory distress, cyanosis of the lips, and her oxygen saturation decreases to 78% on pulse oximetry. No stridor is noted. Lungs are clear to auscultation. An arterial blood gas reveals pH 7.42, PCO_2 40, PO_2 146, oxygen saturation 82%. Which of the following is the most probable diagnosis?

A.   Methemoglobinemia
B.   Pulmonary edema
C.   Laryngospasm

Answer III.17:   A

Pulmonary edema could cause cyanosis and hypoxemia but the clinical exam and PO_2 on ABG are not consistent with this diagnosis. Vocal cords edema, when severe to cause respiratory distress, causes stridor and CO_2 retention.

Methemoglobinemia results from oxidation of ferrous iron to ferric iron within the hemoglobin molecule (1). This molecule cannot bind oxygen and increases the affinity of normal hemoglobin for oxygen, which results in decreased oxygen offloading in the tissues. At elevated levels, methemoglobinemia can cause dyspnea, cyanosis, and even death. The most common finding in all patients is decreased oxygen saturation. There is a disparity between the low oxygen saturation by pulse oximetry and the pO_2 on the arterial blood gas. Common local anesthesia agents such as lidocaine and benzocaine have been correlated with methemoglobinemia (2,3).

In this patient, an overdose of lidocaine (often given via nebulization, nasal spray, instillation through the scope, or nasal gel) was the likely explanation for the signs and symptoms. A high suspicion for methemoglobinemia is required in patients who develop hypoxia or cyanosis after procedures. CO-oximetry can confirm the diagnosis but the clinical picture is often sufficient to proceed with methylene blue treatment or observation, based on how severely the patient is affected. Methylene blue is administered at a dose of 1–2 mg/kg IV slowly over 3–10 minutes (2). In the absence of serious underlying illness, methemoglobin levels less than 30% usually resolve spontaneously over 15–20 hours when the offending agent is removed and oxygen is administered.

References

1. Brown C, Bowling M. Methemoglobinemia in bronchoscopy: a case series and a review of the literature. J Bronchology Interv Pulmonol 2013; 20(3): 241-6.
2. Kwok S, Fischer JL, Rogers JD. Benzocaine and lidocaine-induced methemoglobinemia after bronchoscopy: a case report. J Med Case Rep 2008; 2: 16.
3. Kotler RL, Hansen-Flaschen J, Casey MP. Severe methemoglobinemia after flexible fiberoptic bronchoscopy. Thorax 1989; 44(3): 234-5.

Question III.18: Which one of the following combinations are pharmacological agents of choice for operator-administered sedation in bronchoscopy?

A.   Atropine and Midazolam
B.   Midazolam and Fentanyl
C.   Midazolam and Propofol

Answer III.18:   B

Anti-cholinergic drugs, such as atropine and glycopyrrolate, have been used in the past due to their sympathetic effects which can theoretically prevent vasovagal reactions (bradycardia), reduce coughing and airway secretions during bronchoscopy (1). Clinical trials, however, have failed to demonstrate benefits of these agents in bronchoscopy and their use is not currently recommended.

Benzodiazepines have a long history of safety and efficacy in bronchoscopy and are widely used for sedation. Lorazepam and temazepam have been found to improve patient comfort and willingness to undergo a future procedure, likely due to their amnesic effect. These drugs have now been replaced by midazolam given its rapid onset of action, rapid time to peak effect and short duration of action. The doses used (for sedation) of midazolam, lorazepam and diazepam are 0.01–0.1 mg/kg, 0.03–0.05 mg/kg and 0.04–0.2 mg/kg, respectively.

Opioids are also frequently used in bronchoscopy in combination with benzodiazepines for their analgesic, anti-tussive and sedative properties.

Fentanyl is 100 times as potent as morphine and has a more rapid onset of action and elimination half-life making it more appropriate for use in bronchoscopy. The recommended dose of fentanyl for moderate sedation is 50–200 µg followed by supplemental doses of 50 µg; at the upper limit of this range, however, ventilatory depression is more likely, especially when co-administered with sedatives; therefore, an initial dose of 25–50 µg is recommended with supplemental doses of 25 µg as required until the desired effect is achieved or a total dose of 200 µg has been reached.

Midazolam and a short-acting opioid (i.e. fentanyl) are currently the pharmacological agents of choice for proceduralist-administered sedation in bronchoscopy. Propofol is an anesthetic agent and in many institutions, its administration requires the presence of additional staff knowledgeable (and in many countries, credentialed) in the administration of deep sedation and general anesthesia.

References

1. José RJ, Shaefi S, Navani N. Sedation for flexible bronchoscopy: current and emerging evidence. Eur Respir Rev 2013 ;22(128): 106-16.

Question III.19: A 35-year-old man is brought to the emergency department after a motor vehicle accident. He has respiratory failure and has undergone an emergency tracheotomy. Pneumothorax and four fractured ribs on the right lung are detected on chest radiography. A chest tube was also inserted. There is profuse bleeding from his airways. What other test should be done for the patient?

A.   Diagnostic thoracotomy
B.   Flexible bronchoscopy
C.   Chest magnetic resonance imaging

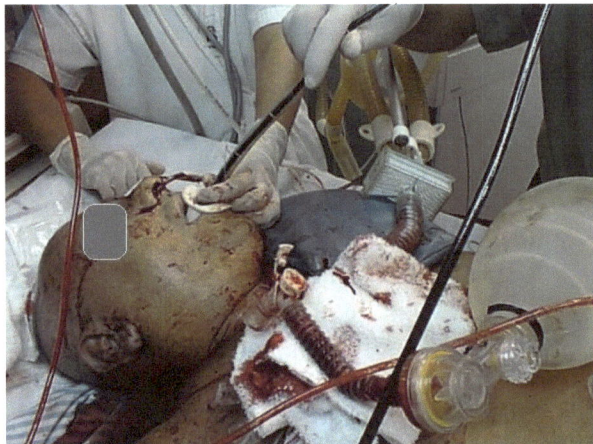

Answer III.19:   B

Airway trauma may be the result of blunt or penetrating injuries to the neck and chest, or of medical procedures that may injure the airway (i.e. endotracheal intubation, especially when emergent or difficult) (1). The presence of concomitant severe body injuries, as well as nonspecific symptoms, may delay the diagnosis and could lead to early mortality or late complications such as airway stenosis and recurrent pulmonary infections.

The symptoms and signs of tracheobronchial injury depend on the site and the severity of the injury and most of them are not specific. Subcutaneous emphysema is the most common finding, occurring in up to 87% of the patients. Pneumothorax occurs in 17-70% of the patients with tracheobronchial injuries. Airway damage is a priority item in the triage/management of trauma victims (2).

These patients should undergo emergency flexible bronchoscopy and careful inspection of the airways to detect and localize a possible tracheobronchial injury. The location, extent, length, and depth of the injury should be noted. Any foreign bodies are removed, and bronchoscopy helps ensure proper endotracheal tube position within the airway (3).

Bronchoscopy in these settings is done while other resuscitation measures are being undertaken. Preserving airway integrity and airway potency, even in the presence of massive airway bleeding can save a life. It is important that bronchoscopists suction blood while preserving ventilation of the contralateral lung and preventing blood from flooding the contralateral airway.

Bronchoscopy often provides a definitive diagnosis in a patient with suspected airway injury. Careful examination of the tracheobronchial tree with the flexible bronchoscope provides information about the location and extent of the injury. In trauma victims with a pneumomediastinum and/or pneumothorax, one must be concerned about possible damage to central airways, especially if: an air leak persists after chest tube insertion, subcutaneous emphysema develops or worsens, signs of tension pneumothorax develop, or the patient develops hemoptysis.

Magnetic resonance imaging is not ideal for imaging the lung parenchyma or airway injuries. In addition, it will not allow the level of minute-to-minute care the patient needs at this time. Thoracotomy may be required after the airway trauma is diagnosed, but this should ideally be offered as a therapeutic, not diagnostic, option after bronchoscopy confirms the diagnosis.

References

1. Prokakis C, Koletsis EN, Dedeilias P, Fligou F, Filos K, Dougenis D. Airway trauma: a review on epidemiology, mechanisms of injury, diagnosis, and treatment. J Cardiothorac Surg 2014; 9: 117.
2. Altinok T, Can A. Management of tracheobronchial injuries. Eurasian J Med. 2014; 46(3): 209-15.
3. Groenendijk MR, Hartemink KJ, Dickhoff C, Geeraedts LM Jr, Terra M, Thoral P, Hashemi SM. Pneumomediastinum and (bilateral) pneumothorax after high energy trauma: Indications for emergency bronchoscopy. Respir Med Case Rep 2014; 13: 9-11.

Question III.20: Which of the following recommendations is true regarding flexible bronchoscopy British Thoracic Society (BTS) guidelines?

A. Only patients with known cardiac disease should have heart rate, blood pressure, and oxygen saturation routinely monitored

B. Oxygen supplementation should be used only when desaturation is significant and prolonged

C. Continuous ECG monitoring should be used for all patients during diagnostic or therapeutic bronchoscopy

D. Coagulation studies, platelet count and hemoglobin levels should be checked in all patients before the bronchoscopy

Answer III.20: B

All patients undergoing bronchoscopy should have heart rate, blood pressure and oxygen saturation recorded repeatedly, including before, during and after the procedure (1). Patients should be monitored by continuous pulse oximetry during bronchoscopy. Oxygen supplementation should be used when desaturation is significant (SpO_2 >4% change and SpO_2 <90%) and prolonged (>1/min) to reduce the risk of hypoxemia-related complications. Continuous ECG monitoring should be used when there is a high clinical risk for arrhythmia. Coagulation studies, platelet count, and hemoglobin should be performed when there are clinical risk factors for abnormal coagulation. Note that options B and C are addressed in the British Thoracic Guidelines (evidence Grade D).

References

1. Du Rand IA, Blaikley J, Booton R, Chaudhuri N, Gupta V, Khalid S, Mandal S, Martin J, Mills J, Navani N, Rahman NM, Wrightson JM, Munavvar M; British Thoracic Society Bronchoscopy Guideline Group. British Thoracic Society guideline for diagnostic flexible bronchoscopy in adults: accredited by NICE. Thorax 2013; 68 Suppl 1:i1-i44.

Question III.21: A 43-year-old man with acute onset of dyspnea, cough and fever was admitted to the ICU for acute hypoxemic respiratory failure. He had symptoms of upper respiratory tract infection one week prior to admission. Post-intubation, arterial blood gas analysis reveals Po_2 60 mmHg, Pco_2 38mmHg, pH 7.432, $PaO_2/FIO_2=100$, PEEP 20 cm H_2O. A chest radiography and computed tomography demonstrate bilateral pulmonary infiltrates. Blood cultures and urine analysis show no evidence of viral, fungal or bacterial infection. Bronchoscopy is performed. A predominance of neutrophils is detected on bronchoalveolar lavage (BAL) cell count and differential. No ventricular dysfunction and no evidence of increased pulmonary arterial or right ventricular pressure is noted on echocardiography. A diagnosis of Acute Respiratory Distress Syndrome (ARDS) is made on clinical criteria and the patient receives supportive care following the low tidal volume ventilation protocol. Given the lack of a predisposing factor for (ARDS), which of the following is the most probable diagnosis?

A.   Cryptogenic organizing pneumonia
B.   Acute hypersensitivity pneumonitis
C.   Acute interstitial pneumonitis

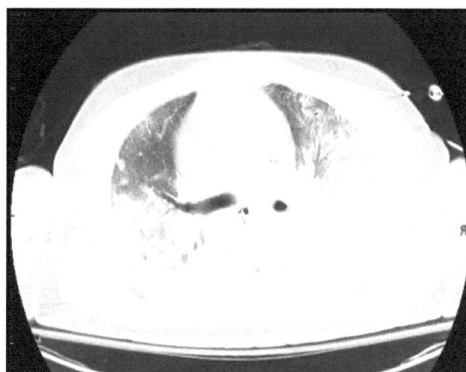

Answer III.21:   C

The term acute interstitial pneumonitis (AIP) is used for cases previously named Hamman-Rich syndrome, reflecting an acute form of idiopathic interstitial lung disease (1). The criteria for a diagnosis of AIP include acute onset of respiratory symptoms resulting in severe hypoxia and, in most cases, acute respiratory failure, bilateral lung infiltrates on radiographs, the absence of an identifiable etiology or predisposing condition despite the adequate clinical investigation and histological documentation of diffuse alveolar damage (DAD).

This patient met all criteria except for the histologic one, as biopsy was not performed during the procedure (high risk for pneumothorax given high PEEP). AIP is characterized histologically by diffuse alveolar damage, a histopathologic pattern that includes hyaline membranes, alveolar exudates, and microthrombi. DAD is the underlying histologic pattern of approximately 60% of cases of ARDS. Mortality is high (30% to 40%) but returns to near-normal respiratory function is possible in survivors.

AIP is often preceded by a viral-like or flulike prodromal illness or upper respiratory tract infection characterized by fatigue and myalgias, followed by acute onset of dyspnea and cough, accompanied by fever, in some cases. Most patients suffering from AIP present with hypoxia on room air, and the majority require mechanical ventilation. Radiographically, the presence of bilateral lung infiltrates varies from patchy to diffuse. Because AIP is defined as an idiopathic entity, known causes of DAD need to be excluded before the term AIP is applied.

Infection, therefore, must be excluded in patients with a diagnosis of AIP. This should take the form of microbiological and serological testing, including cultures of sputum, blood, bronchial washings, and/or bronchoalveolar lavage (BAL) fluid. The BAL in AIP has a predominance of neutrophils (2). AIP is indistinguishable from ARDS by BAL or surgical lung biopsy. It is typically steroid-unresponsive. Treatment is supportive.

References

1. Mukhopadhyay S, Parambil JG. Acute interstitial pneumonia (AIP): relationship to Hamman-Rich syndrome, diffuse alveolar damage (DAD), and acute respiratory distress syndrome (ARDS). Semin Respir Crit Care Med 2012; 33(5): 476-85.
2. Schwarz MI, Albert RK. "Imitators" of the ARDS: implications for diagnosis and treatment. Chest 2004; 125(4): 1530-5.

Question III.22: Which of the following statements is correct regarding the diagnostic role of bronchoscopy in non-HIV-infected immunocompromised patients with lung infiltrates?

A.   The diagnostic yield is higher for infectious than for noninfectious causes
B.   BAL has a better diagnostic yield than transbronchial lung biopsy (TBLB)
C.   BAL with TBLB and BAL alone have similar diagnostic yields

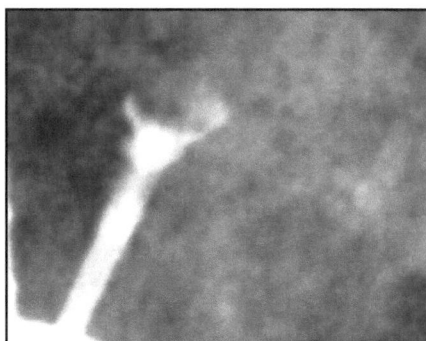

Answer III.22:   A

At least one prospective observational study evaluated the diagnostic role of flexible bronchoscopy (FB) in immunocompromised patients with pulmonary infiltrates (1). The study population consisted of 104 consecutive non-HIV-infected immunocompromised patients with lung infiltrates. The overall diagnostic yield of FB was 56.2% (95% confidence interval [CI], 47 to 64%). FB provided at least one diagnosis in 53 of 104 patients (51%; 95% CI, 40 to 62%). FB was more likely to establish the diagnosis when the lung infiltrates were due to an infectious agent (81%; 95% CI, 67 to 90%) than to a noninfectious process (56%; 95% CI, 43 to 67%; p = 0.011). The diagnostic yields of BAL (38%; 95% CI, 30 to 47%) and TBLB (38%; 95% CI, 27 to 51%) were similar (p = 0.94). The diagnostic yield of brushing was lower (13%; 95% CI 6 to 24%; p = 0.001) than that of BAL. The combined diagnostic yield of BAL and TBLB (70%; 95% CI, 57 to 80%) was higher than that of BAL alone (p < 0.001). Also, the diagnostic yield of FB with brushing, BAL, and TBLB was similar to that of FB with BAL and TBLB. The complication rate from FB was 21% (95% CI, 15 to 31%). Minor bleeding (13%) and pneumothorax (4%) were the most common complications.

The authors concluded that FB is a procedure of choice for identifying the cause of lung infiltrates in non-HIV immunocompromised patients. Since BAL and TBLB are complementary, unless contraindications exist, it is warranted to perform TBLB whenever it is deemed safe (risks and benefits of biopsy must be carefully weighed) because it adds to the diagnostic yield. In contrast, brushings added no value to BAL and TBLB.

References

1. Jain P, Sandur S, Meli Y, Arroliga AC, Stoller JK, Mehta AC. Role of flexible bronchoscopy in immunocompromised patients with lung infiltrates. Chest 2004; 125(2): 712-22.

Question III.23: A 34-year-old man presents with a 5-day history of fever and dyspnea. He has a recent diagnosis HIV infection and antiviral therapy has not been initiated yet. The CD4 count and viral load are pending. A regimen of broad-spectrum antibiotics is started, but his dyspnea is worsening. Oxygen saturation is 96% with FIO_2 of 70%. A chest radiograph shows bilateral reticulonodular infiltrates. Bronchoscopy is performed. BAL smear showed alveolar macrophages with numerous intracellular yeast-like organisms with eccentric chromatin. What is the likely diagnosis?

A. Tuberculosis
B. Actinomycosis
C. Histoplasmosis

Answer III.23:   C

The BAL findings describe the dimorphic fungus Histoplasma capsulatum (1). The clinical manifestations of histoplasmosis vary from asymptomatic to severe disseminated disease. The majority of patients present with respiratory symptoms. Acute histoplasmosis is usually a self-limiting disease, with fever, chills, nonproductive cough, headaches, and generalized malaise. Disseminated histoplasmosis (DH) is usually encountered in newborns and immunocompromised patients, especially those with acquired immunodeficiency syndrome (AIDS). The most frequent manifestations in DH patients are fever (95%), cough (75%), weight loss (72%), diarrhea (61%) and fatigue (56%) (1). Acute renal failure, respiratory insufficiency, and septic shock can be seen in DH patients.

Diagnosis is made on the isolation of *H. capsulatum* by culture, fungal stains of tissue or body fluids, and tests for antibodies and antigens. Although bone marrow biopsy and culture have the highest diagnostic yield, BAL specimen and culture is also used for diagnosis (2). *H. capsulatum* may be recovered from sputum, BAL fluid, or lung tissue in up to 70% of cases (3).

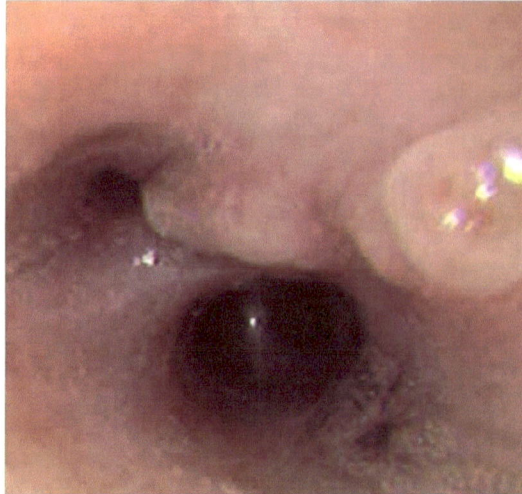

Example of endobronchial
Histoplasmosis

References

1. Daher EF, Silva GB Jr, Barros FA, Takeda CF, Mota RM, Ferreira MT, Oliveira SA, Martins JC, Araújo SM, Gutiérrez-Adrianzén OA. Clinical and laboratory features of disseminated histoplasmosis in HIV patients from Brazil. Trop Med Int Health 2007; 12(9): 1108-15.
2. Valdivia-Arenas MA, Sood N. A 77-year-old farmer with respiratory failure and thrombocytopenia. Chest 2006; 129(5): 1378-81.
3. Vathesatogkit P, Goldenberg R, Parsey M. A 27-year-old HIV-infected woman with severe sepsis and pulmonary infiltrates. Disseminated histoplasmosis with severe sepsis and acute respiratory failure. Chest 2003; 123(1): 272-3, 274-6.

Question III.24: A 45-year-old Caucasian male from California (USA) is admitted to the MICU for respiratory distress. He has cough and fever at admission and is HIV-positive. A chest radiography shows bilateral reticulonodular infiltrates and mediastinal adenopathy. Bronchoscopy is performed. Erythema and narrowing of the lower lobe bronchi are observed (See Figure below). Diff–Quik stain on an EBUS-TBNA sample shows granulomas in the subcarinal and right paratracheal lymph nodes. Bronchoalveolar lavage (BAL) reveals thick-walled spherules containing endospores. What is the diagnosis?

A.   Pulmonary Tuberculosis
B.   Disseminated Coccidioidomycosis
C.   Pulmonary Actinomycosis
D.   Disseminated Histoplasmosis

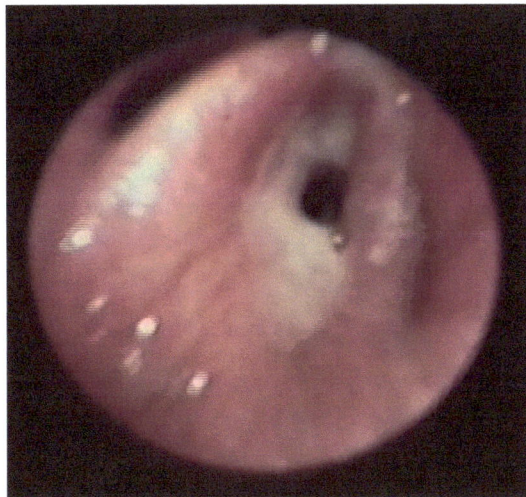

Answer III.24:   B

Coccidioidomycosis results from inhaling the spores of Coccidioides immitis. Most infections in the United States occur within the endemic regions: southern Arizona, central California, southern New Mexico, and west Texas (1). Risk factors for this infection are HIV infection, organ transplant, pregnancy, diabetes mellitus and the use of infliximab (2). The majority of immunocompetent people exposed are either asymptomatic but some may develop an influenza-like illness and occasionally pneumonia (2). Dissemination is uncommon in immunocompetent hosts. Bronchoscopy is used for diagnosis.

Endobronchial Coccidioidomycosis may show airway erythema (3). Invasive procedures, such as bronchial brushing or lavage, with fungal smear and culture, or biopsy, may be needed to confirm the diagnosis. A lymph node biopsy can also show granulomas or granulomatous inflammation. Fungal stains could show the spherules and surrounding inflammation.

The organisms most commonly encountered in granulomatous inflammation of the lung are mycobacteria and fungi (4). The most common fungal causes of pulmonary granulomas are Histoplasma, Cryptococcus, Coccidioides, and Blastomyces. Prevalence of these fungi varies by geographic region. In the United States, Histoplasma is primarily seen in the central and eastern states, Coccidioides is endemic in the Southwest, Cryptococcus is ubiquitous, and Blastomyces in the Great Lakes basin.

References

1. Galgiani JN, Ampel NM, Catanzaro A, Johnson RH, Stevens DA, Williams PL. Practice guideline for the treatment of Coccidioidomycosis. Infectious Diseases Society of America. Clin Infect Dis 2000; 30(4): 658-61.
2. Rogan MP, Thomas K. Fatal miliary Coccidioidomycosis in a patient receiving infliximab therapy: a case report. J Med Case Rep 2007; 1: 79.
3. Polesky A, Kirsch CM, Snyder LS, LoBue P, Kagawa FT, Dykstra BJ, Wehner JH, Catanzaro A, Ampel NM, Stevens DA. Airway Coccidioidomycosis--report of cases and review. Clin Infect Dis 1999; 28(6): 1273-80.
4. Mukhopadhyay S, Gal AA. Granulomatous lung disease: an approach to the differential diagnosis. Arch Pathol Lab Med 2010; 134(5): 667-90.

Question III.25: A 25-year-old man with AIDS is suspected of having tuberculosis. Three sputum samples show no acid-fast bacilli on smears. The patient has a cough productive of minimal whitish-yellowish thick mucus. Bronchoscopy is considered by the treating team as a next step in this patient's management but the bronchoscopy team is concerned about being exposed to multi-drug resistant tuberculosis. Which of the following should be considered to confirm tuberculosis in this patient?

A.   Pre-bronchoscopy sputum culture
B.   Post-bronchoscopy sputum culture
C.   Bronchoalveolar lavage culture

Answer III.25:   A

Patients with HIV infection have a lower sensitivity of sputum smear for acid-fast bacillus (AFB). As a result, the prevalence of smear-negative tuberculosis is on the rise in HIV-infected patients. The diagnostic yield of pre- and post-bronchoscopy sputum and bronchoalveolar lavage (BAL) in sputum smear-negative, HIV-positive patients was evaluated in one study (1). *Mycobacterium tuberculosis* was isolated from 21.7%, 19.7% and 15.3% of BAL, post- and pre-bronchoscopy sputum cultures, respectively. Acid-fast stain (AFS) on pre-bronchoscopy sputum using concentration technique and direct AFS on BAL together detected 41% of the culture-positive cases. In patients who could produce sputum, the sensitivity of pre-bronchoscopy sputum culture (15.3%) was comparable to BAL (14%) and post-bronchoscopy sputum (14%). In patients who could not produce sputum, however, both BAL (40%) and post-bronchoscopy sputum (31.4%) detected significantly more patients than those who could produce sputum (P=0.002, P=0.028, respectively).

It appears that in HIV-infected patients, AFS by concentration method on pre-bronchoscopy sputum and direct AFS on BAL in patients who cannot produce sputum are the preferred methods of making a rapid diagnosis. BAL culture seems to add little value in patients who can produce sputum; therefore, bronchoscopy could be deferred under such circumstances. It is noteworthy that sputum induction using hypertonic saline is often warranted, although some patients (up to a fifth in one study) may still be unable to provide a sample (2).

References

1. Aderaye G, G/Egziabher H, Aseffa A, Worku A, Lindquist L. Comparison of acid-fast stain and culture for Mycobacterium tuberculosis in pre- and post-bronchoscopy sputum and bronchoalveolar lavage in HIV-infected patients with atypical chest X-ray in Ethiopia. Ann Thorac Med 2007; 2(4): 154-7.
2. Peter JG, Theron G, Singh N Et al. Sputum induction to aid diagnosis of smear-negative or sputum scarce tuberculosis in adults in HIV-endemic settings. Eur Respir J 2014; 43:185-194.

Question III.26: The routine performance of coagulation studies, platelet or hemoglobin is of little or no value in predicting bleeding after bronchoscopic lung biopsy.

A. True
B. False

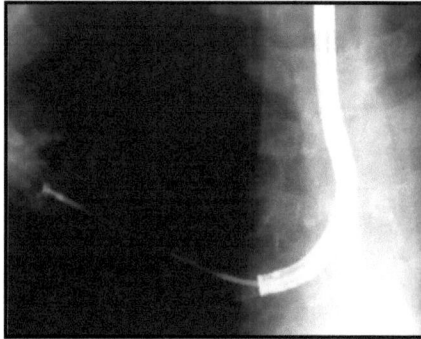

Answer III.26:   A

The routine performance of coagulation studies, platelet or hemoglobin is of little or no value in predicting bleeding after bronchoscopic lung biopsy (1). These should be performed when there are clinical risk factors for abnormal coagulation. Bronchoalveolar lavage (BAL) can be performed with platelet counts >20 000 per µL. Platelet transfusion may be necessary before bronchoscopy if an endobronchial biopsy (EBB) or TBLB will be performed.

References

1. Du Rand IA, Blaikley J, Booton R, Chaudhuri N, Gupta V, Khalid S, Mandal S, Martin J, Mills J, Navani N, Rahman NM, Wrightson JM, Munavvar M; British Thoracic Society Bronchoscopy Guideline Group. British Thoracic Society guideline for diagnostic flexible bronchoscopy in adults: accredited by NICE. Thorax 2013; 68 Suppl 1:i1-i44.

Question III.27: Bronchoscopy on noninvasive ventilation is preferred to elective intubation for diagnostic purposes. This statement is

A. True
B. False

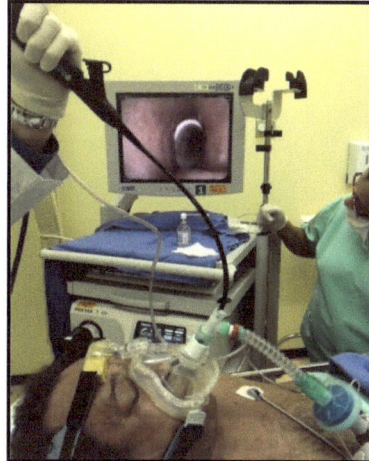

Answer III.27:   A

      Bronchoscopy on noninvasive ventilation is preferred to elective intubation for bronchoscopy purposes because it can avoid intubation-associated risks such as aspiration, ventilator-associated pneumonia, ventilator-associated lung injury and airway injury (1).

References

1. Murgu SD, Pecson J, Colt HG. Bronchoscopy during noninvasive ventilation: indications and technique. Respir Care 2010; 55(5): 595-600.

Question III.28: Which of the following is most likely to be beneficial immediately in a patient with increasing tachypnea, oxygen desaturation, and the chest radiograph below?

A. Postural drainage and supplemental oxygen
B. Chest physical therapy
C. Flexible bronchoscopy

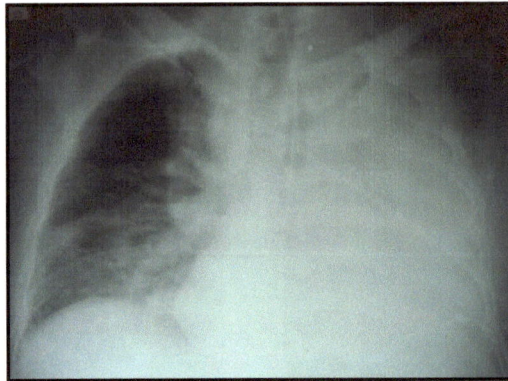

Answer III. 28:   C

Flexible bronchoscopy with inspection and aspiration of secretions can resolve atelectasis, as well as make a diagnosis. Saline washing allows removal of mucus plugs blood or thick secretions. Subsequent chest physical therapy, postural drainage, and supportive care with early mobilization will assist in preventing recurrent atelectasis. Bronchoscopy will also help detect underlying causes of central airway obstruction such as a tumor, benign diseases, or foreign bodies that may block the central airways and prompt lobar or complete lung atelectasis.

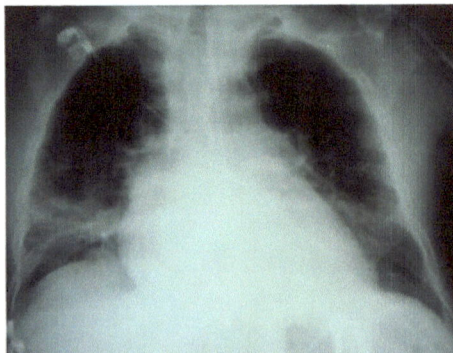

After bronchoscopic removal of
thick secretions and mucus plugs.

Question III.29. A fifty-year-old male presents to the emergency department with severe tachypnea and hemoptysis. A flexible bronchoscopy is performed revealing near-total tracheal obstruction from what appears to be a large adenoma (see Figure below). You are called to evaluate the patient for admission to the intensive care unit. What is your next step?

A. Admit the patient to the ICU. Ask for anesthesia, thoracic surgery, and interventional pulmonology consultation.

B. Keep the patient in the seated or upright position. Immediately request anesthesia, thoracic surgery and interventional pulmonology consultation with a request for probable awake intubation over the flexible bronchoscope in the emergency department or operating theater and/or immediate therapeutic bronchoscopy.

C. Move the patient to radiology for an immediate computed tomography scan

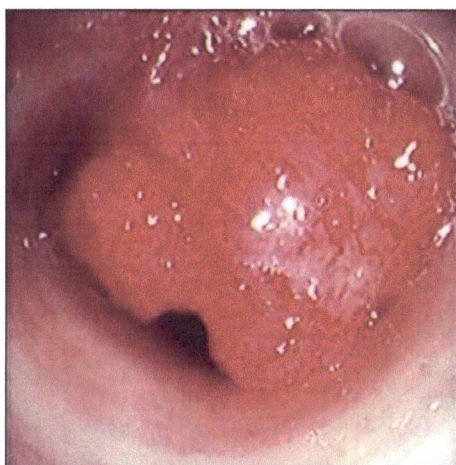

Photo courtesy L. Oto

Answer III.29:   B

     This patient has significant risk for complete airway obstruction, respiratory failure, and death. It is also likely that he has retained secretions or blood in the airways distal to the obstruction. His condition, therefore, represents an emergency best handled either by careful endotracheal intubation under direct bronchoscopic guidance, and/or immediate transfer to the operating theater for bronchoscopic resection. Keeping the patient seated helps maintain airway patency (versus the reclined position). Keeping the patient awake and not sedated helps retain his capacity to cough in order to clear secretions as needed.

     Resectional techniques might include flexible or rigid bronchoscopy, Nd:YAG laser resection, cryo-resection, argon beam, or electrocautery. Careful technique will be required to avoid significant bleeding and further airway obstruction. It is likely this tumor can be removed in toto, although it may be necessary to insert an airway stent, which might be placed at the time of the initial procedure, or at a later date if needed. After the procedure, the patient is best served by hospitalization in the intensive care unit for further stabilization.

Airway potency restored following bronchoscopic resection. Photo obtained from distal margin of the resection.

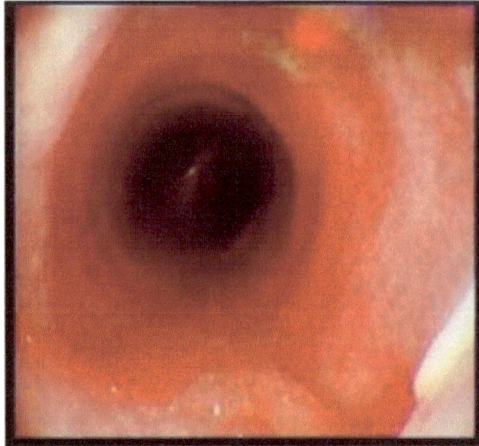

Photo courtesy L. Oto

Question III.30. A 72-year-old woman with unresectable esophageal cancer is admitted to the Intensive Care Unit with bilateral lower lobe pulmonary infiltrates, and suspected aspiration pneumonia based on history. She also reports increasing difficulty swallowing. This is the second time in three weeks that she is admitted to the hospital, and her condition appears to be worsening. You decide to perform flexible bronchoscopy as part of the critical care evaluation. The finding below is most consistent with:

A. Esophageal-airway fistula from necrosing esophageal cancer
B. Left main bronchial mass
C. Mediastinal adenopathy and tuberculosis eroding into the airway

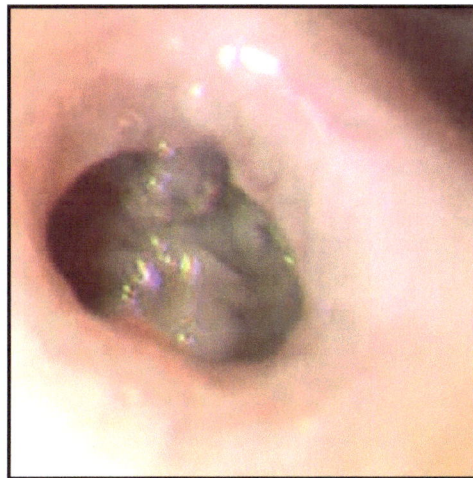

Answer III.30:   A

The image is most consistent with a necrosing esophageal cancer eroding into the airway. Recurrent aspiration is a frequent symptom, and if the tumor is impinging on the esophagus, will also cause increasing dysphagia. Prior radiation therapy is the most common risk factor for esophago-respiratory fistulas. Palliative treatment might include insertion of an esophageal stent, and in some cases, insertion of both an esophageal and airway stent depending on symptoms, and whether there is evidence of central airway obstruction (1-5). The image does not show an endobronchial mass. Mediastinal adenopathy from Tuberculosis can erode into the airway, especially at the level of the carina and subcarina, but usually, there is evidence of white, creamy, caseating material and a history of tuberculosis.

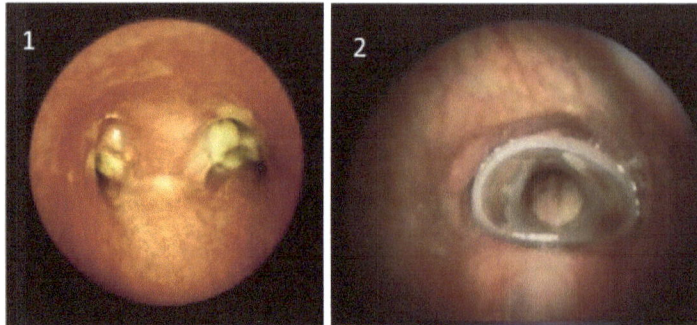

(1) Tuberculous lymphadenopathy eroding through main carina. (2) Tracheal silicone stent used to occlude tracheo-esophageal fistula

References

1. Mingyao Ke, Xuemei Wu, and Junli Zeng. The treatment strategy for tracheoesophageal fistula. J Thorac Dis. 2015 Dec; 7(Suppl 4): S389–S397.
2. Colt HG, Meric B, Dumon JF. Double stents for carcinoma of the esophagus invading the tracheobronchial tree. Gastrointest Endosc.1992;38:485–489.
3. Fabrice Paganin, Laurent Schouler, Laurent Cuissard, et al. Airway and Esophageal Stenting in Patients with Advanced Esophageal Cancer and Pulmonary Involvement. PLoS ONE. 2008; 3(8): e3101. Published online 2008 Aug 29. doi: 10.1371/journal.pone.0003101.
4. Lenz CJ, Bick BL, Katzka D, et al. Esophagorespiratory Fistulas: Survival and Outcomes of Treatment. J Clin Gastroenterol. 2016 Nov 7. [Epub ahead of print]
5. Bick BL, Song LM, Buttar NS, et al. Stent-associated esophagorespiratory fistulas: incidence and risk factors. Gastrointest Endosc. 2013 Feb;77(2):181-9. doi: 10.1016/j.gie.2012.10.004. Epub 2012 Dec 11.

***

CONGRATULATIONS

You have now completed Module III of The Essential Intensivist Bronchoscopist©.

The following section contains a ten question post-test and answers.

Post-tests are True/False. Please remember that while many programs consider 70% correct responses a passing grade, the student's "target" score should be 100%.

Please send us your opinion regarding Bronchoscopy Education Project materials by contacting your national bronchology association or emailing us at
www.bronchoscopy.org.

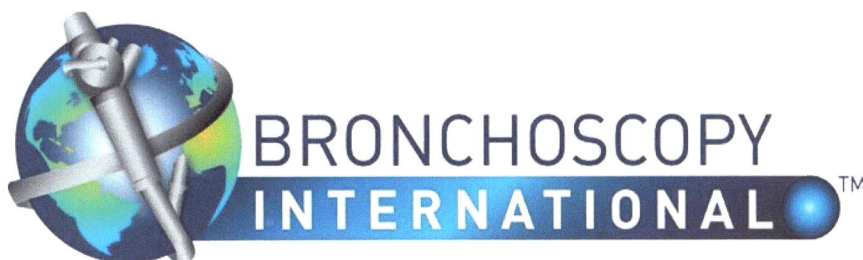

MODULE III

TEN QUESTION TRUE/FALSE POST-TEST

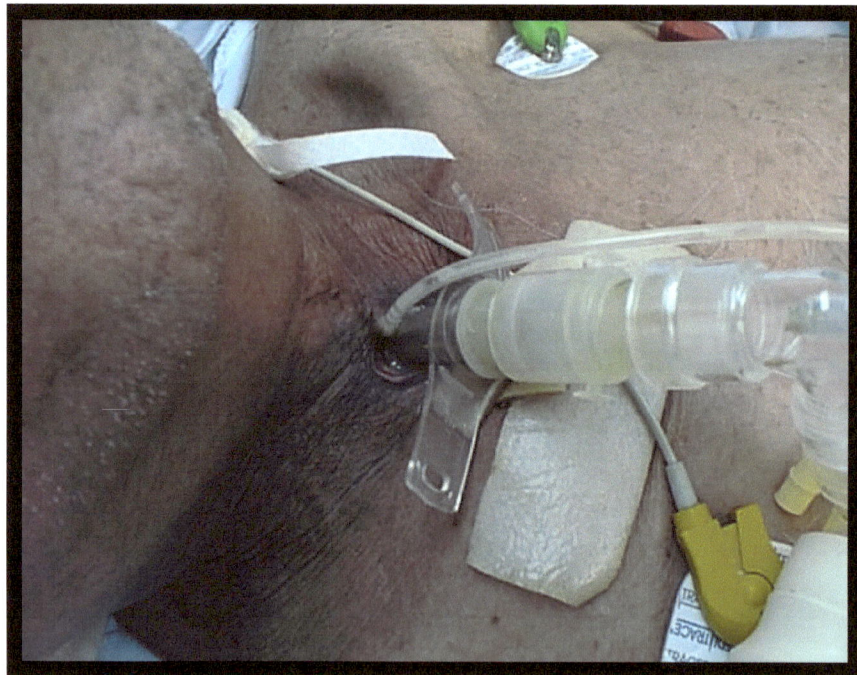

The Essential Intensivist Bronchoscopist

Module III Post-test

INSTRUCTIONS: Answer True or False to each of the following <u>TEN</u> questions.

Question 1: Bronchoscopy is expected to change management decisions in approximately 50% of patients with neutropenia and pulmonary infiltrates.

Question 2: Bronchoscopy can be expected to provide diagnostic information in more than 60% of oncologic patients with acute respiratory failure.

Question 3: Results from several studies show that quantitative cultures of BAL fluid and nonquantitative cultures of endotracheal bronchial aspirates in patients with ventilator-associated pneumonia result in similar clinical outcomes.

Question 4: Bronchoscopy may reveal acute lung injury, infection, colonization, airway strictures, or rejection in up to 70% of critically ill lung transplant recipients.

Question 5: Results of BAL can be expected to change antimicrobial treatment in more than 50% of patients with fever, hematologic malignancy, and pulmonary infiltrates.

Question 6: Lidocaine overdose-related seizures (as part of bronchoscopy topical anesthesia) is most likely in critically ill elderly patients with liver disease.

Question 7: Clopidogrel should be stopped at least 5-7 days prior to bronchoscopy with bronchoalveolar lavage in critically ill patients.

Question 8: Fentanyl and midazolam are choice agents for moderate sedation in critically ill patients because of their rapid onset of action, rapid time to peak effect, and short duration of action.

Question 9: Flexible bronchoscopy is warranted in all patients with suspected or witnessed inhalation injury.

Question 10: HIV positive patients have similar sensitivity of sputum smears for acid-fast bacilli as non-HIV patients.

***

Answers to

The Essential Intensivist Bronchoscopist post-test Module III

ANSWERS

1. True
2. False
3. True
4. True
5. False
6. True
7. False
8. True
9. False
10. False

TOTAL SCORE _____/10

MODULE IV

THIRTY MULTIPLE CHOICE QUESTION/ANSWER SETS

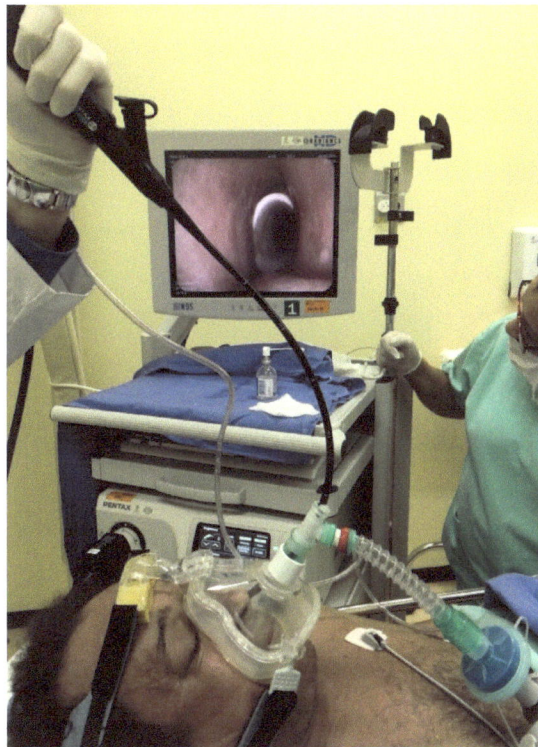

The Essential Intensivist Bronchoscopist©

The Essential Intensivist Bronchoscopist MODULE IV

LEARNING OBJECTIVES

After completing this module the reader should be able to:

1. Describe at least three complications of bronchoscopic intubation.
2. List the indications for bronchoscopy in inhalation and burn victims and describe at least three possible bronchoscopic findings with subsequent management.
3. Enumerate five rules for evaluating patients with a known or suspected difficult airway.
4. Describe all four classes of the Mallampati score.
5. Describe at least five laryngeal or subglottic airway abnormalities that might represent a difficult airway warranting awake intubation or deployment of a specialized multidisciplinary difficult airway management team.

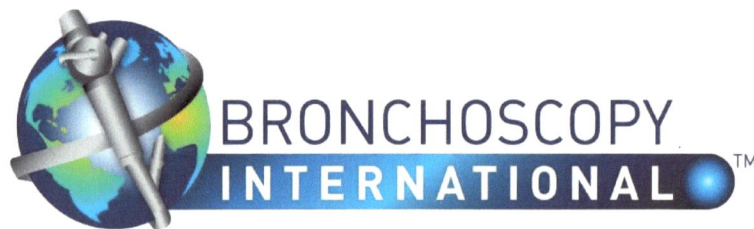

BRONCHOSCOPY INTERNATIONAL™

Question IV.1: While intubating a patient over the flexible bronchoscope, you are unable to advance the endotracheal tube because it is repeatedly caught on the larynx. The tip of the bronchoscope is in the midtrachea and you are able to visualize normal appearing vocal cords upon scope insertion. Which of the following is the best maneuver to proceed with successful intubation?

A. Withdraw the bronchoscope from the trachea and into the endotracheal tube. Repeat an attempt at intubation.
B. Without moving the flexible bronchoscope, withdraw the endotracheal tube slightly, then rotate it 90 degrees counterclockwise or clockwise in order to reverse the locations of its beveled end and Murphy eye. Then gently advance the tube again.
C. Ask your assistant to withdraw the endotracheal tube while you maintain the bronchoscope in position directly below the vocal cords. This straightens the tube so that intubation can be reattempted.

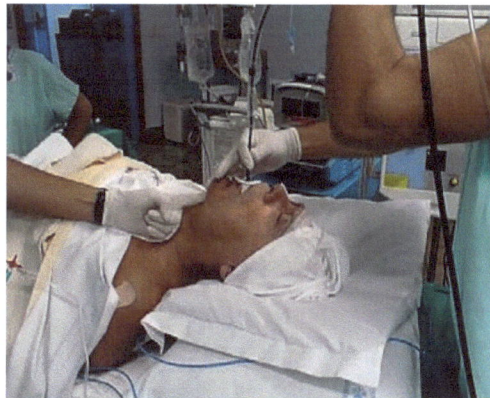

Answer IV.1: B

Asking an assistant to manipulate the endotracheal tube is always a risk because it may be accidentally displaced, resulting in removing both the tube and the bronchoscope from the airway. Positioning the bronchoscope in the immediate subglottis might also increase the risk of losing the airway, and you might never visualize the cords again. Intubation could then become impossible, especially if blood, secretions, redundant tissues, or reflex laryngospasm impairs visualization.

As long as the bronchoscope is in the lower airways, even if intubation is delayed, oxygen can be delivered directly through the working channel of the bronchoscope into the trachea to prevent hypoxemia. The opportunity for this potentially life-saving gesture is lost if the scope is removed from the trachea.

The best alternative is to keep the flexible bronchoscope in position within the trachea. Withdrawing the endotracheal tube slightly moves it off the larynx. Subsequent, gentle rotation of the endotracheal tube 90 degrees clockwise or counterclockwise, changes the place of the bevel tip and Murphy eye. This alters the angle of entry and allows an easier advancement of the endotracheal tube over the scope. Remember to lubricate the bronchoscope prior to inserting it into the endotracheal tube.

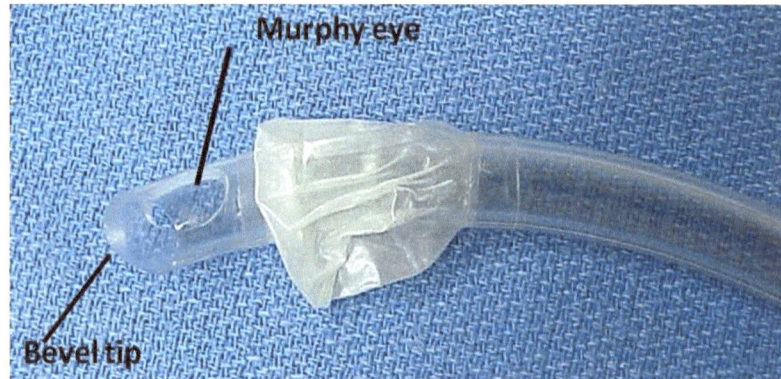

Question IV.2: Several days after a difficult intubation and mechanical ventilation, extubation is performed over the flexible bronchoscope. During removal, you inspect the upper airways. The abnormality you see represents:

A. A subluxation of the right arytenoid
B. Trauma-related edema of the right arytenoid
C. Laryngeal swelling from laryngeal cancer

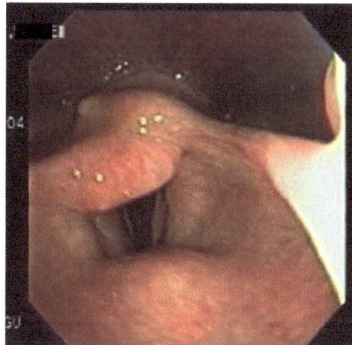

Answer IV.2:   A

This image (figure a) represents a subluxation of the right arytenoid, a rare but possible complication of intubation, and one that if pre-existing can make intubation difficult. This highlights the importance of performing a careful bronchoscopic examination of the upper airway and laryngeal structures prior to attempting intubation over the bronchoscope. Other complications that may occur as a consequence of intubation include a swollen epiglottis and arytenoids (figure b) and left vocal cord ulceration (figure c). Vocal cord paralysis in the median position should be identified if present. Note that after extubation, laryngeal dysfunction often lasts up to four hours. Additional possible consequences of extubation also place patients at risk for reintubation: patients with airway obstruction, hypoventilation syndrome, hypoxic respiratory failure, unprotected airway and aspiration, and retained secretions requiring pulmonary hygiene.

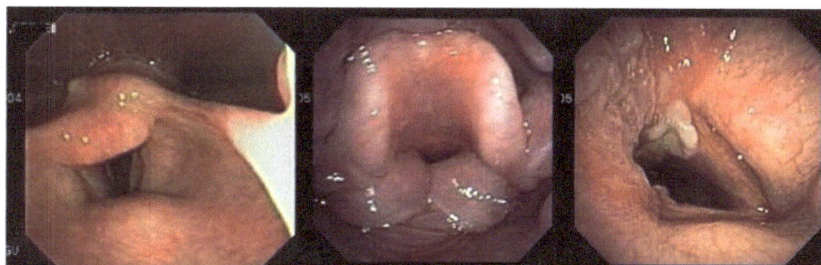

Figure a.   Figure b.   Figure c.

Question IV.3: Emergency intubation is required in an awake adult male trauma victim with a neck brace and restricted cervical spine mobility. The patient's tongue is swollen, and he is spitting blood from a laceration of the lower lip. After clearing the oropharynx of blood and secretions using a Yankauer suction cannula, which of the following actions is <u>best</u>?

A. Intubate the patient using an oral approach and a 7.0 endotracheal tube over a small diameter (4.8mm) flexible bronchoscope.
B. Intubate the patient using a nasal approach, a 6.0 mm flexible bronchoscope, and an 8.0 endotracheal tube.
C. Intubate the patient using a nasal approach, a 6.0 mm flexible bronchoscope, and a 7.5 endotracheal tube.

Answer IV.3:   **C**

Repeated attempts at intubation are often unsuccessful and traumatic. Precious time is wasted and the risks for hypoxemia are increased. Therefore, it is wise to succeed with intubation at the first attempt. Although not ideal, emergency nasal intubation usually provides ready access to the larynx and establishment of an emergency airway. The nares serve as a splint that guides the bronchoscope toward the larynx. In addition, this technique avoids risks associated with potential mobility or cervical spine movement. Endotracheal tubes can, if necessary, be replaced at a later date, either in the Intensive Care Unit or in the operating suite in a more controlled setting. During intubation, it may help to grasp the patient's tongue with a gauze pad, and to ask an assistant to pull the tongue out of the mouth slightly. This creates more space to maneuver in the oropharynx. Gentle insertion of the endotracheal tube over a flexible bronchoscope in an awake patient helps avoid reflex laryngospasm, reflex arrhythmias, vomiting, and the risks of over sedation in a patient with an unstable or not yet existent airway.

A well lubricated, larger diameter bronchoscope with a larger diameter suction channel might be important in a patient with abundant secretions or blood. This also allows better control of the endotracheal tube than a small diameter bronchoscope. By filling up more of the space within the endotracheal tube, the larger-sized scope and endotracheal tube are more readily maneuverable. Although it is generally recommended to intubate with the largest size endotracheal tube possible, most experts agree that a 7.5 endotracheal tube is the largest diameter tube that should be inserted through the nares. Some experts use a combination of the nasal approach using a small diameter bronchoscope and endotracheal tube, with a second operator handling a laryngoscope. The second operator can thus aspirate the airways, and potentially facilitate endotracheal tube insertion using, for example, Magill forceps.

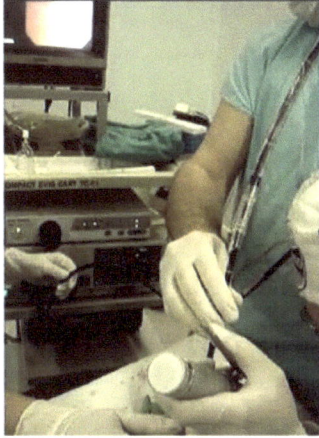

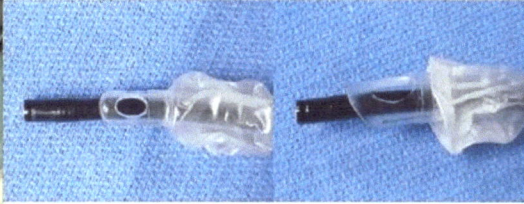

Space between #8 endotracheal tube and flexible bronchoscope. There is no space between the scope and a #6 endotracheal tube

A second person may use laryngoscopy to assist with endotracheal tube insertion.

References

1. Branson RD, Gomaa D, Rodriguez D Jr. Management of the artificial airway. Respir Care 2014;59:974-989.

Question IV.4: A 67 year old male diagnosed with adult onset asthma four years earlier is admitted to the Intensive Care Unit for cough and moderate dyspnea unresponsive to inhaled bronchodilators. He has a moderate wheeze on auscultation over the trachea but has good lung sounds and shows little accessory muscle use. He speaks hesitantly and follows commands. A chest radiograph obtained in the Emergency Department revealed an intratracheal shadow. After obtaining a computed tomography scan, the best plan of action is to:

A. Sedate and oxygenate, then perform flexible bronchoscopy for airway inspection followed by appropriate referral to thoracic surgery and/or interventional pulmonology
B. Refer to an interventional pulmonary specialist for bronchoscopic evaluation and bronchoscopic resection
C. Call anesthesia and prepare for rapid sequence intubation

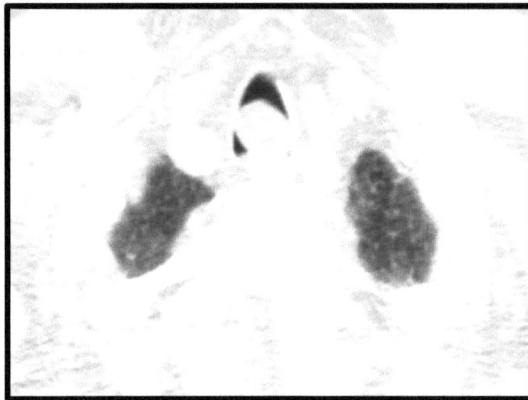

Answer IV.4:   B

The CT scan shows an intratracheal mass completely obstructing airway lumen. The mass is likely obstructing the lumen intermittently (ball-valve effect) because the patient speaks hesitantly and is in only moderately dyspneic, suggesting good air entry, but poor exhalation. Referral to a specialist for bronchoscopy and possible resection or intubation in a controlled environment, depending on bronchoscopic appearance and suspected diagnosis is preferable to emergency endotracheal intubation in this stable patient. Sedation prior to inspection bronchoscopy in the ICU risks the complete loss of airway.

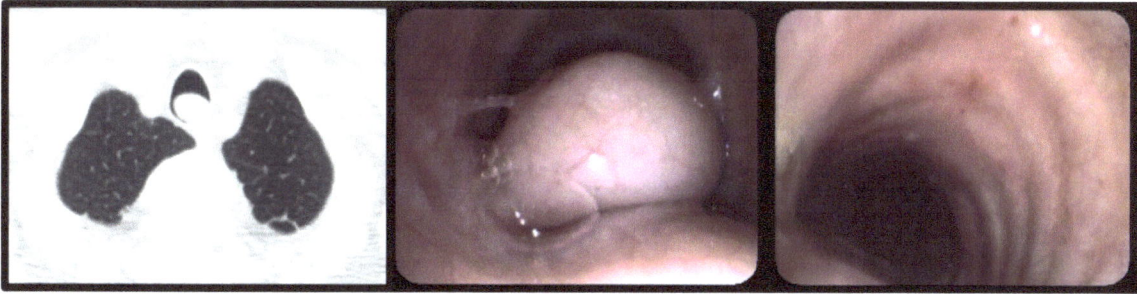

Intratracheal lipoma resected using electrocautery snare under rigid bronchoscopy.

References

1. Catalanotti V, Bertaglia V, Tariq N et al. Ball valve effect as a cause of acute respiratory failure during palliative chemotherapy for small cell lung cancer. J Cancer Biol and Research 2014;2:1035-1036.

Question IV.5:   Propofol has been associated with hypotension, respiratory depression, metabolic acidosis, and anaphylactic shock. Intravenous administration of short-acting, perioperative intravenous Propofol, however, does NOT cause which of the following?

A. Bradycardia
B. Analgesia
C. Psychosis

Answer IV.5:   B

Propofol is a hypnotic-sedative, anticonvulsant, and amnestic frequently used in the operating theater, minimally invasive procedure suite, intensive care unit, and endoscopy/bronchoscopy suite. Its onset of action is within 30-60 seconds of intravenous administration. Its duration of action is 5-15 minutes. While its respiratory depression and hypotensive effects are well known, it may also cause metabolic acidosis, arrhythmias, anaphylactic shock, rhabdomyolysis with and renal failure, skin rash, and liver failure. There are reports of acute psychosis. It is not an analgesic. Propofol is also an ideal agent for rigid bronchoscopy.

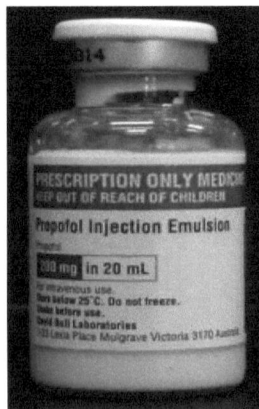

References

1. Perrin G, Colt HG, Martin C et al. Safety of interventional rigid bronchoscopy using intravenous anesthesia and spontaneous assisted ventilation: a prospective study. Chest 1992;102:1526-1530.

Question IV.6: After performing bronchoscopy through the endotracheal tube, you were able to visualize the carina and distal airways. It suddenly becomes difficult to remove the bronchoscope. What happened?

A. The bending tip of the bronchoscope broke.
B. The tip of the bronchoscope has accidentally passed through the Murphy eye of the endotracheal tube.
C. The polyurethane covering of the bronchoscope has broken, occluding the endotracheal tube lumen.

Answer IV.6:   B

This accident can occur during bronchoscopy as well as while performing bronchoscopic intubation over the bronchoscope. Before intubating over a bronchoscope, one should make sure the bronchoscope is functioning correctly. Passage of the tip of the bronchoscope through the Murphy eye of the endotracheal tube is avoided by fully loading and keeping the endotracheal tube high on the scope prior to intubation. During bronchoscopy, one should be aware of any changes in angulation or resistance as the scope is passed through the endotracheal tube. If the bronchoscope is caught inside the Murphy eye, and cannot be dislodged by gentle rotation, it may be necessary to remove both the scope and the endotracheal tube simultaneously, after which the patient must be reintubated. Rupture of the polyurethane cover is very rare and would usually not obstruct visualization. When the tip of a bronchoscope breaks, it usually becomes unmaneuverable and goes into a neutral position that still allows feeding an endotracheal tube over it.

After loading the endotracheal tube high onto the bronchoscope, note the radio-opaque markers on the endotracheal tube, as well as the direction of the Murphy eye and distal opening of the endotracheal tube. Some experts believe that the endotracheal tube should remain fully loaded onto the bronchoscope until the tip of the scope is passed well beyond the vocal cords. The endotracheal tube is then fed into the trachea using the Seldinger technique.

Other experts recognize that on some occasions, such as when there is subglottic stenosis, laryngeal edema, tumor, a tracheal stent, blood, or secretions, it might be preferable to keep the tip of the bronchoscope inside the endotracheal tube. The bronchoscope-endotracheal tube ensemble is then passed simultaneously past the cords. In case of severe tracheal stenosis, this technique avoids blind, forceful dilation of the stricture because the bronchoscopist sees and feels the tube pass through the stenosis.

Intubation techniques should be practiced on inanimate models. The bronchoscopist should use the technique with which he or she is most experienced, and always choose the safest technique based on the patient's underlying illness and ventilatory status.

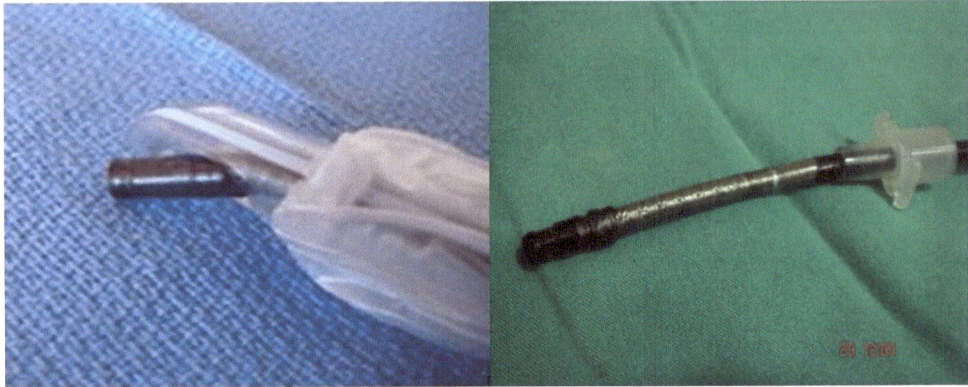

Endotracheal tube through Murphy eye
results in destroyed bronchoscope sheath

Question IV.7: Which of the following suggests <u>inappropriate</u> indications for flexible bronchoscopy in an intensive care unit?

A. Bronchoscopy is performed frequently in critically ill patients with atelectasis, copious secretions, and elevated airway pressures while on mechanical ventilation.
B. Bronchoscopy is performed frequently in critically ill patients with new onset of hemoptysis.
C. Bronchoscopy is performed frequently in critically ill patients with copious secretions but no radiographic evidence of atelectasis.

Answer IV.7:   C

Bronchoscopic practice varies according to available resources, staffing, institutional and individual biases, and referring physician preferences. If, however, numerous procedures are being performed without clear indications, or if bronchoscopy does not affect medical management, the reasons for excess bronchoscopic procedures should be explored in order to ensure patient safety, ethical clinical practice, and cost-effective medical care delivery. Numerous studies have shown the benefit of chest physiotherapy, which in many instances can be done instead of bronchoscopy to help mobilize and remove secretions from critically ill, mechanically ventilated patients. Bronchoscopy, therefore, is usually reserved for patients with radiographic abnormalities such as atelectasis or pulmonary infiltrates, or when copious secretions and mucous plugs may increase airway resistance and peak airway pressures.

In addition to performing bronchoscopy for hemoptysis or recurrent atelectasis in critically ill patients, indications for bronchoscopy in the intensive care unit include but are not limited to include copious secretions that cannot be cleared by routine suctioning, persistent or acute unexplained hypoxemia, unexplained failure to wean from mechanical ventilation, persistent recurrent hemoptysis, pulmonary infiltrates with suspicion for infection when the bronchoscopic procedure is likely to alter therapy, persistent or hemodynamically significant radiographic atelectasis that is unresponsive to chest physical therapy or suctioning, emergency or controlled intubation, pre-lung transplant airway evaluation, suspicion of expiratory central airway collapse, and to assist diagnosis in patients who are difficult to wean from mechanical ventilation.

References

1. Fragoso GC, Goncalves GM. Role of fiberoptic bronchoscopy in intensive care unit: current practice. J Bronchol Intervent Pulmonol 2011;18:69-83.

Question IV.8: Bronchoscopy is performed in a critically ill adult patient with impending respiratory failure. Which of the following is suggestive of expiratory central airway collapse?

A. The tracheal transverse diameter is decreased by 10% (about 2 mm) during expiration
B. The tracheal transverse diameter is decreased by 80 % during expiration
C. The tracheal sagittal diameter is decreased 20% during expiration

Answer IV.8:   B

     The cross-sectional shape of the trachea is characterized by the ratio of transverse (separates trachea into front and back) and sagittal (separates trachea into left and right) diameters. Women tend to preserve a round configuration, while men tend to have some sagittal widening and transverse narrowing. Usually, there should be no significant change in tracheal sagittal diameter during normal expiration because surrounding negative intrathoracic pressure supports airway patency. It is important to evaluate these patients without positive pressure ventilation if possible, and very slight sedation. In non-intubated patients, forced expiratory maneuvers and coughs can be performed at the completion of an examination in order to better evaluate the existence, location, extent, degree, and type of expiratory central airway collapse.

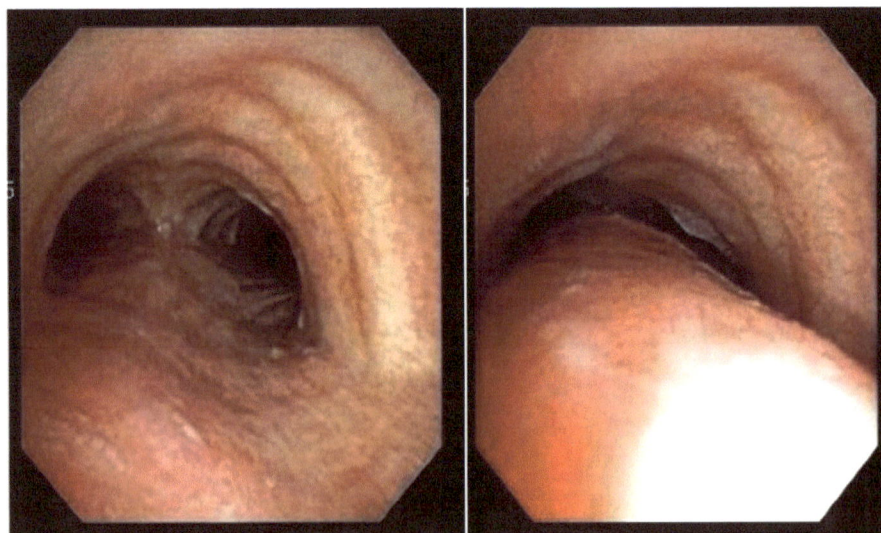

Inspiration   Expiration

Question IV.9: Which of the following pulmonary function disturbances is prompted by bronchoscopy in a mechanically ventilated patient?

A. Reduced functional residual capacity
B. Reduced positive end-expiratory pressure
C. Increased airway resistance

Answer IV.9:   C

Airway resistance is increased because the cross-sectional area of the trachea, usually about 3 cm^2, is reduced by the endotracheal tube and by the flexible bronchoscope within the endotracheal tube. End-expiratory pressure and functional residual capacity are actually increased because of the increase in airway resistance. Procedures should be continued cautiously or stopped if peak airway pressures increase significantly, or if bronchoscopy causes hypertension, significant tachycardia, dysrhythmias, or significant oxygen desaturation. If possible, a flexible bronchoscope should not occupy more than 60% of the endotracheal tube lumen (which usually means using a bronchoscope with an external diameter 2mm less than the internal diameter of the tube).

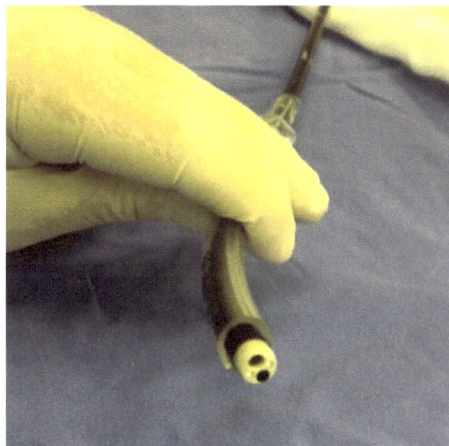

Question IV.10: The image showed most likely demonstrates:

A. Paralyzed vocal cords in abduction
B. Subglottic tracheal stenosis
C. Normal vocal cords are seen through the tracheostomy stoma from below

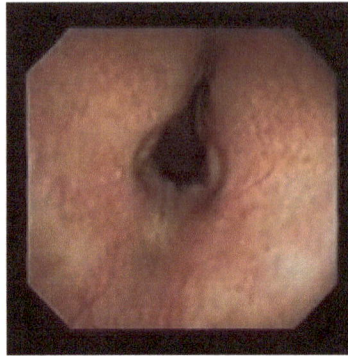

Answer IV.10   C

The image is that of the vocal cords seen through the stoma from below. The flexible bronchoscope was introduced through the tracheostomy, after removing the tracheotomy tube. The scope is flexed cephalad in order to examine the subglottis. The patient is asked to phonate. Here, normal vocal cords are seen in abduction. The subglottis is normal. Indications for this procedure include suspected subglottic or parastomal source of bleeding, and inspection of the subglottis for cartilaginous abnormality, stricture, or to fully evaluate laryngeal function prior to removal of a tracheostomy tube.

Question IV.11: Which of the following statements about inhalation injury is <u>correct</u>?

A. Parenchymal damage is often delayed for hours or even days.
B. Airway edema and laryngeal swelling are reliable indicators of parenchymal lung injury
C. Intubation is warranted only if airway edema and soot are noted on bronchoscopy

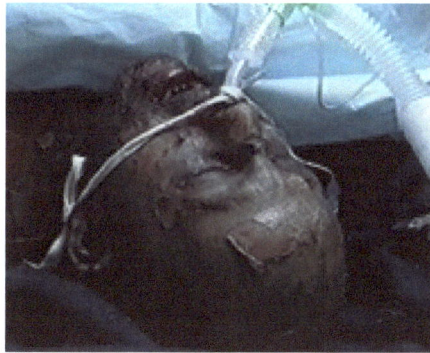

Answer IV.11:   A

Airway mucosal findings, chest radiographs, and arterial blood gases are notoriously unhelpful in predicting whether parenchymal injury or further airway damage has occurred after inhalation injury. For these reasons, in many burn centers, all smoke exposed victims, including those who asymptomatic, are closely monitored in the ICU. Bronchoscopy is indicated if there is the slightest doubt of airway involvement, and in many burn centers, is performed routinely, especially in case of symptoms. In most cases, the presence of airway edema, mucosal swelling, or soot provides direct evidence of heat damage and inhalation injury, in which case many specialists recommend intubation and mechanical ventilation. Radiographic abnormalities and oxygenation problems may be delayed hours and even days. In addition, maximum upper airway edema peaks as late as 36-48 hours after injury, prompting many experts to bronchoscopically monitor patients with early signs of airway injury. The presence of dyspnea, wheezing, laryngeal abnormalities, tracheobronchitis, and abnormal arterial blood gases or chest radiographs almost always warrants intubation. Delayed problems include tracheobronchial tissue sloughing, decreased mucociliary clearance, mucous plugging, atelectasis, impaired clearance of secretions, pneumonia, pulmonary edema and acute respiratory distress syndrome.

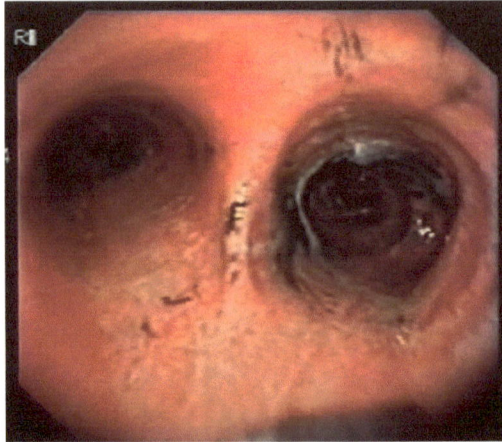

Soot, hyperemia, and edema from inhalation injury

References

1. Kim Y, Kym D, Hur J et al. Does inhalation injury predict mortality in burns patients or require redefinition? PLoS One 2017;12:30185195.
2. Walker PF, Buehner MF, Wood LA et al. Diagnosis and management of inhalation injury: an updated review. Crit Care 2015;19:351.

Question IV.12: Which of following statements about bronchoscopy in burn victims is <u>correct</u>?

A. The evidence of airway injury in smoke inhalation and cutaneous burn victims rarely affects prognosis compared to cutaneous burn injury alone
B. Bronchoscopic findings consistent with inhalation injury in burn victims are usually airway edema, inflammation, or carbonaceous secretions (presence of soot)
C. Erythema, hemorrhage, and ulceration are rare manifestations of airway injury in burn victims

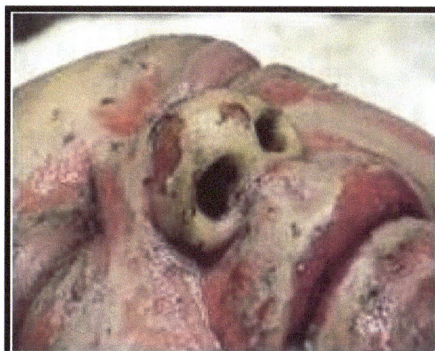

Answer IV.12:   B

Erythema, hemorrhage, and ulcerations are frequently noted as a direct effect of thermal injury to the upper or lower airways. In burn victims, inhalation injury significantly increases mortality when compared to cutaneous burn injury alone. This occurs most frequently from hot smoke or steam inhalation. In fact, the use of bronchoscopy for diagnosis in suspected inhalation injury victims (based on history, carbonaceous sputum, and facial burns) has resulted in a recognized increase in the incidence of inhalation injury to as high as 30 percent incidence.

The upper airway protects the lower airway and parenchyma, and any exposures to hot air may cause reflex laryngospasm. Edema and inflammation are proof of upper airway injury and are often immediately visible to the bronchoscopist. Laryngeal complications can occur acutely, as well as many hours after injury. They are frequently life-threatening.

While the presence of carbonaceous secretions in the oropharynx suggests airway damage, lower airway injury is typically delayed. Therefore, some experts suggest that immediate intubation in patients with suspected injury is preferred to a watch and wait approach. The presence and extent of lower airway injury are usually ascertained by monitoring patients with serial bronchoscopies.

In patients who were intubated in the field or upon hospital admission, extubation is usually delayed until all edema has resolved. Intubation and mechanical ventilation may be extended because of persistent laryngeal and subglottic edema, or swelling due to the endotracheal tube. The absence of endotracheal tube leak, airway edema or airway strictures at the time of bronchoscopically-guided extubation is helpful indicators of a successful extubation.

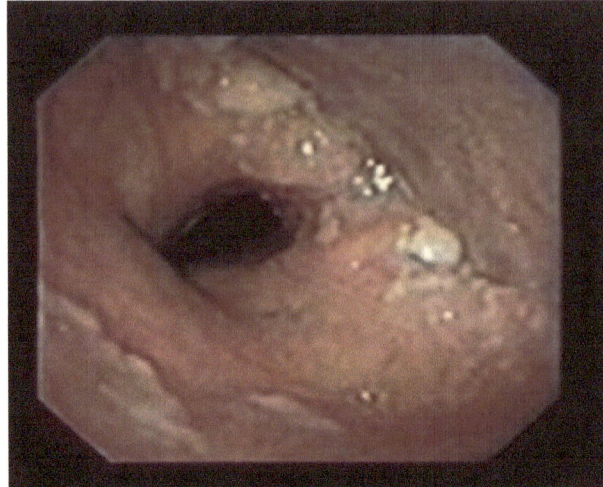

Thermal injury and laryngeal edema
in a burn/inhalation injury victim

References

1. Spano S, Hanna S, Li Z, et al. Does bronchoscopic evaluation of inhalation injury severity predict outcome? J Burn Care Res 2016;37:1-11.

Question IV.13: Which of the following statements about moderate sedation is <u>correct</u>?

A. Moderate sedation is always warranted in critically ill patients requiring bronchoscopy
B. Moderate sedation relieves patient anxiety but may prompt respiratory failure in patients with impending respiratory insufficiency.
C. Topical lidocaine is unnecessary in critically ill, intubated and moderately sedated patients.

Answer IV.13:   B

      Although bronchoscopy without sedation is safe, most bronchoscopists believe that short-acting moderate sedation should be offered to help improve patient comfort. The benefits of moderate sedation (anxiety relief, amnesia, analgesia, improved cooperation) should always be weighed against its disadvantages (need for additional monitoring, risk of respiratory depression, and risk of decreased patient cooperation because of inhibitions or restlessness). Topical anesthetic decreases airway reactivity and cough, and should, therefore, be administered even in intubated and mechanically ventilated patients.

      In certain instances, procedures without sedation may be warranted in a fully awake and cooperative individual. Possible indications include patients with hemoptysis or foreign body when a conscious cough may be helpful, and patients requiring dynamic bronchoscopy and in whom controlled breathing exercises help diagnose causes of expiratory central airway collapse. Patients being extubated over the flexible bronchoscope can also undergo the procedure without sedation, even when a complete airway inspection is performed prior to extubation. Sedation can also be avoided in patients on the verge of respiratory failure and in whom intubation must be avoided (patients with advance directives prohibiting intubation and mechanical ventilation, for example). In these cases, bronchoscopy using continued positive airway pressure is a consideration.

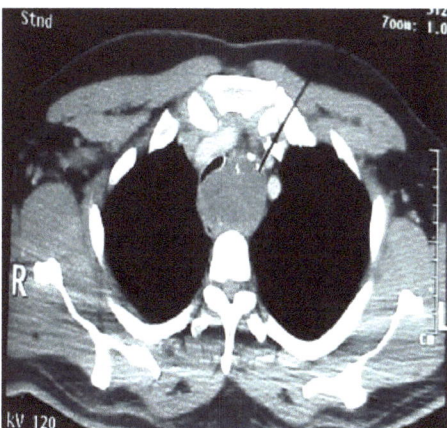

Many experts would avoid sedation if performing inspection bronchoscopy in this patient with a large paratracheal tumor (prior to emergent referral for stent insertion) because sedation may contribute to and exacerbate respiratory insufficiency. Ideally, the procedure should probably be performed with the patient in a seated position.

Question IV.14: Which of the following is usually an early complication of tracheostomy tubes?

A. Tracheo-innominate artery fistula
B. Tracheo-esophageal fistula
C. Tracheomalacia

Answer IV.14:   A

Tracheo-innominate artery fistula is usually an early complication of tracheostomy tube insertion and is reported in as many as 0.7 % of patients with a tracheotomy. About 50% of patients with this complication of tracheotomy have a sentinel bleed before massive hemorrhage age (1). Treatment usually requires a median sternotomy. Malacia is usually a later finding, sometimes due to chronic infection and cartilaginous damage. Tracheoesophageal fistula can occur both early and late in the course of hospitalization and is reported in as many as 0.5 % of patients with a tracheostomy. Cough, hemoptysis, or dyspnea in patients with a history of tracheotomy should always prompt bronchoscopy in order to identify airway abnormalities potentially responsible for symptoms.

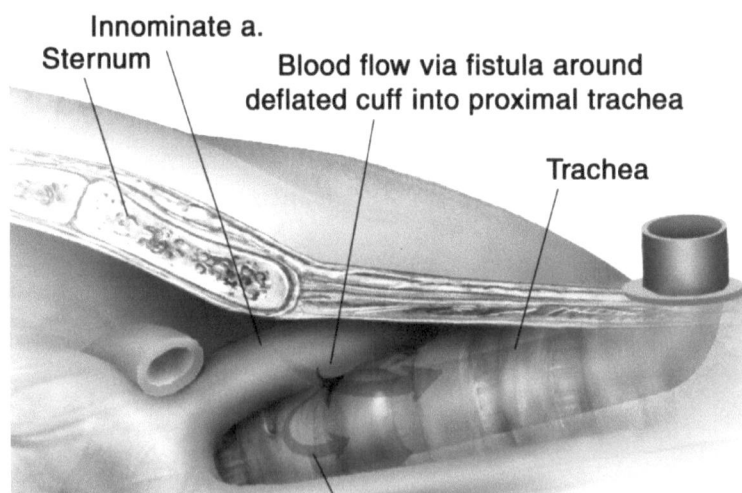

From Aliawade G, downloaded from Elsevier Science Direct, April 9, 2017

References

1. Aliawadi G. Technique for managing tracheo-innominate artery fistula. Operative Techniques for Thoracic and Cardiovascular Surgery 2009; 14;66-72.

Question IV.15: Which of the following drugs consistently suppresses airway reflexes and is therefore considered most beneficial for awake tracheal intubation?

A. Midazolam
B. Diazepam
C. Fentanyl

Answer IV.15:   C

Midazolam, Diazepam, and Fentanyl are used for moderate sedation. Large doses of each of these drugs can also produce general anesthesia and suppress all reflexes. Fentanyl, however, is usually preferred over midazolam or diazepam in patients requiring awake intubation because of its faster action and shorter duration of action. It is noteworthy that Propofol, another choice for patients requiring an awake intubation, is a hypnotic-sedative that also suppresses airway reflexes.

Fentanyl is a synthetic opiate analog 100 times more potent than morphine. Given intravenously, its onset of action is within 2 minutes of injection. Its maximum respiratory depression effect occurs 5-10 minutes after injection, and the effect lasts anywhere from 30-60 minutes. Fentanyl is structurally different from morphine or meperidine. The usual adult dose is 50-100 micrograms. Given intramuscularly, the onset of action is within 7-15 minutes with a duration of action lasting up to two hours. Fentanyl should be avoided in patients receiving MAO inhibitors because of increased risk of respiratory depression and coma.

References

1. https://www.webmd.com/drugs/2/drug-6253/fentanyl-transdermal/details/list-interaction-details/dmid-1480/dmtitle-fentanyl-maois/intrtype-drug.

Question IV.16: The anatomic structure shown in the Figure below is:

A. The most narrow part of the adult male airway
B. The most narrow part of the adult female airway
C. The most narrow part of the pediatric airway

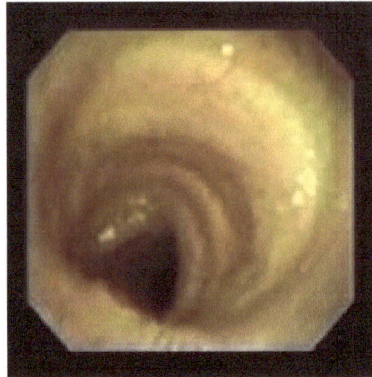

Answer IV.16:   C

The cricoid is the narrowest part of the pediatric airway. The glottis is the narrowest part of the adult airway. In children, the epiglottis and larynx are usually more anterior than in adults, and the trachea is more easily collapsible. A child's oral tissues and mucous membranes are often floppy in the mouth and pharynx.

In case of intubation, uncuffed endotracheal tubes are usually used in children under age 8. The external diameter of the endotracheal tube should approximate the size of the child's nares. Better still to use a Broselow tape measure usually available in most emergency rooms.

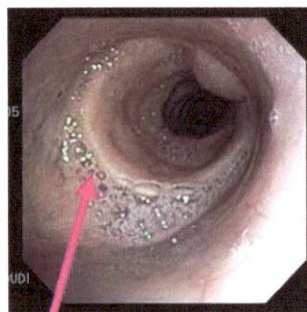

Cricoid cartilage

Question IV.17: A 29-year-old woman with Polyangiitis granulomatosis (GPA previously known as Wegener's granulomatosis) and increasing shortness of breath undergoes emergency flexible bronchoscopy. Based on this finding shown you should.

A. Attempt to pass the bronchoscope beyond the subglottic stricture in order to measure its length.
B. Request an endotracheal tube at the bedside, then attempt to push the bronchoscope beyond the stricture to examine the remaining airway and determine whether the stricture is simple or complex.
C. Stop the examination, remove the bronchoscope. Keep the patent under observation, and urgently notify otolaryngology, thoracic surgery and an interventional bronchoscopist of the finding.

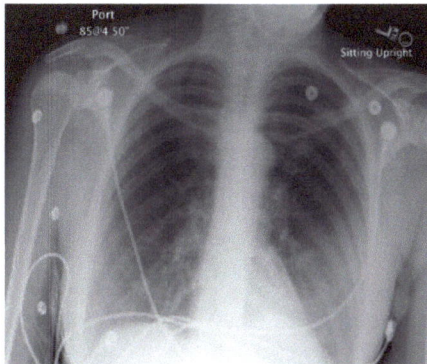

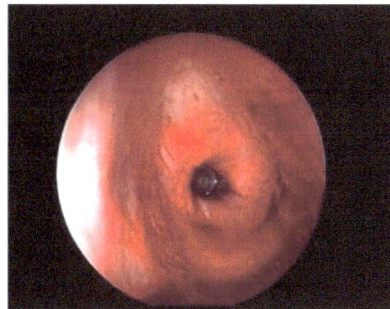

Answer IV.17:   C

Continuing the bronchoscopic examination or attempting to dilate the stricture is dangerous. Remember to "never take away something you cannot give back". It is wiser to continue the evaluation in the hands of an experienced interventional bronchoscopist able to organize a multidisciplinary approach to this patient's airway problem and systemic vasculitis.

Although limited GPA may involve only the subglottis, usually causing firm subglottic narrowing, it may also involve the upper and even the entire trachea as well as lobar and segmental bronchi. Overall, less than 10 percent of patients with GPA are believed to have tracheobronchial involvement.

This severe subglottic stricture is life-threatening. In addition, it appears that the patient has had an indwelling stent placed in the subglottic stricture and that the stent has migrated distally. It is important for all patients with airway stents to have a medical alert document in their possession. This document states the location of the stricture and type of stent inserted.

The stent can be drawn in the location on the schematic of the airway (Downloadable from The Bronchoscopy International website (stent alert document).

Medical Alert
My Airway Stent

Name_____

Size: Diameter   Length

Location: Subglottis   Trachea

Left main bronchus   Right main bronchus
Tracheobronchial

PATIENTS! Contact Dr. XXX or his staff

Weekdays (xxx) xxx-xxxx, xxx-xxxx

After hours call (xxx) xxx-xxxx

Have operator page Doctor on call

OR go to the nearest ER if you have

- New or increased shortness of breath
- New or increased chest pain
- New or increased cough or hemoptysis
- New or increased hoarseness or loss of voice

DOCTORS! Potential complications of airway stents include migration, obstruction by secretions, obstruction by tissue growth or tumor, infection and atelectasis.

- Most stents can be seen on chest radiographs as "straight lines".
- Emergent intubation can be performed using a cuffless #6 endotracheal tube.
- Urgent flexible bronchoscopy may be warranted.

Medical alert document for airway
stent patients (www.Bronchoscopy.org)

References

1. Dutau H, Dumon JF. Airway stenting revisited: 30 years, the age of reason? J Bronchol and Intervent Pulmonol 2017;24:257-259.
2. Girard C, Charles P, Terrier B et al. Tracheobronchial stenoses in granulomatosis with polyangiitis (Wegener's). Medicine 2015;94:e1088

Question IV.18: A 43-year-old woman with a history of healed tracheostomy is admitted to the intensive care unit after being clinically stabilized in the emergency department. She is wearing oxygen via nasal canula. She has tachypnea and audible stridor. While preparing for flexible bronchoscopy you:

A. Administer intravenous sedation and heliox
B. Place the patient's head and neck in the "sniff" position
C. Administer mist humidification

Answer IV.18:   B

The sniff position is frequently the first step required to improve passage through the upper airways, glottis, and subglottis. Originally described in 1913 by Chevalier Jackson, the sniff position is reached by simply placing a small pad under the patient's head for adults (1). This extends the cervical vertebrae at the atlantoaxial joint and flexes the lower cervical vertebral joints. However, at least one study shows it does not always prompt three axis alignment (oral-pharyngeal and laryngeal). Additional jaw elevation results in extension of the head and forward projection of the base of the tongue. Placing a pad that is too large can hinder maximal mouth opening.

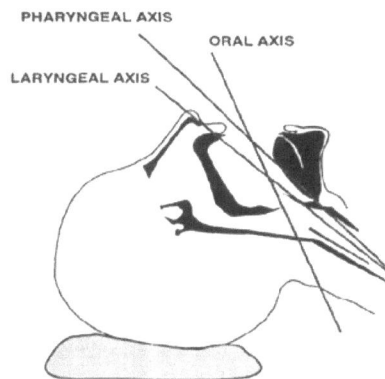

Presumed alignment of oral, pharyngeal,
and laryngeal axes by sniff position
Downloaded from: https://airwayjedi.com/2016/04/01/positioning-the-head-for-intubation/

References

1. Adnet F, Borron SW, Lapostolle F et al. The three-axis alignment theory and the "sniffing position": perpetuation of an anatomic myth? Anesthesiology 1999;12:1964-1965.

Question IV.19: Which of the following statements is <u>correct</u> about approximate airway dimensions?

A. The usual distance between of the orifice of the right upper lobe bronchus and the main carina is about 2 cm.
B. The usual length of the left main bronchus is 4-5 cm. It bifurcates sharply from the midline of the trachea at an angle of 70 degrees.
C. The usual length of the right main bronchus is 1.0 cm. It bifurcates at an angle of 25 degrees from the midline of the trachea.

Answer IV.19:   A

The right main bronchus is 2 cm long on average (not 1 cm as suggested in response C), and has an internal diameter of 10-16 mm. This is slightly larger than the diameter of the left main bronchus. Because the right main bronchus is relatively straight and vertical, aspiration into this bronchus is more frequent than on the left. The left main bronchus is much longer than the right main bronchus. It is usually 4-5 cm long and bifurcates from the main carina at an angle of about 45 degrees (not 70 degrees as suggested in response B). These distances are important to know in case of right or left main bronchial selective intubation and of course in case of placement of bronchial blockers for selective ventilation or management of airway bleeding.

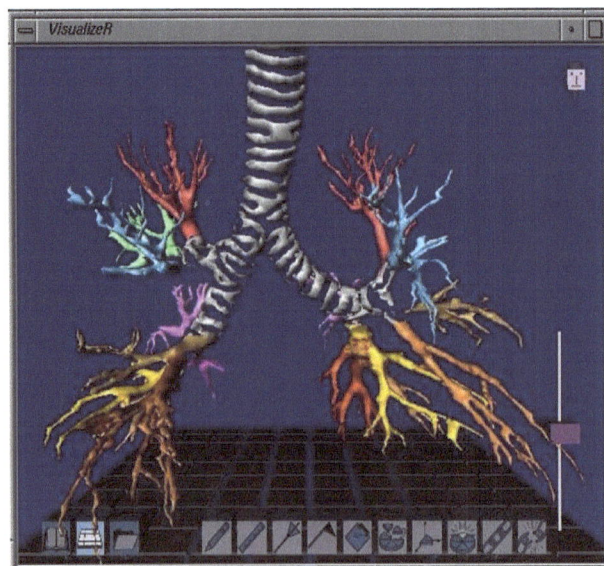

Question IV.20: Which of the following statements about endotracheal intubation is correct?

A. The female's glottis opening and tracheal cross-sectional area are smaller than a male's. Therefore, smaller endotracheal tubes can usually be used in women
B. Cricoid pressure is dangerous in both men and women at risk of aspiration
C. Patients with heart failure, myocardial ischemia or hypovolemia provide no additional risk of peri-intubation mortality compared to patients without such comorbidities.

Answer IV.20:   A

An adult woman's glottis is usually smaller than that of a man (on average a woman's rima glottidis (the middle space between the vocal cords) is 12 mm in diameter with maximum abduction of the white vocal folds (1). A man's vocal folds are usually thicker than a woman's, and in full abduction noticed if the patient is asked to inhale deeply; the man's glottic opening is larger (on average about 19 mm).

The average cross-sectional area of the male adult trachea is approximately 2.8 cm^2. The average cross-sectional area, as well as tracheal length, diameter and volume correlate with body height. In adults, the average cross-sectional area at age 30 is about 2.8 cm^2, increasing to an average of approximately 3.2 cm^2 by age 60. The cross-sectional area of a female is about 40 percent less than that of a male.

Cricoid pressure is safely performed in men and women at risk of aspiration. The presumed goal of cricoid pressure is to collapse the esophagus between the cricoid cartilage and the spine. This prevents passive aspiration of gastric contents during induction of anesthesia, rapid sequence intubation, and resuscitation when intubation is delayed or not possible. Multiple specialty societies, however, report that cricoid pressure is not effective in preventing aspiration during or before rapid sequence intubation, and may actually worsen laryngoscopic visualization as well as impair bag-valve-mask ventilation.

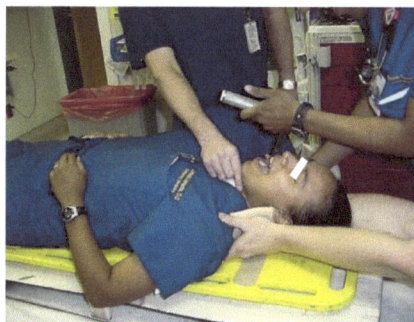

References

1. Stewart JC, Bhananker S, and Ramaiah R. Rapid-sequence intubation and cricoid pressure. Int J Crit Illn Inj Sci. 2014 Jan-Mar; 4(1): 42–49.

IV.21: Complications related to airway management are most frequent in which of the following settings?

A. Operating theater
B. Outpatient setting
C. Intensive care unit

Answer IV.21:   C

According to several studies, complications related to airway management are most frequently encountered in the ICU setting. For example, in one study from difficult airways and arrhythmias were encountered in 12% and 10% respectively in the ICU as compared to 4% and 0.8% in the operating room (1). In addition to competently performing the procedure, responsibilities of bronchoscopists in the ICU include team leadership, knowing how to evaluate and manage patients with a difficult airway, developing a plan for each procedure that includes being prepared for all possible airway or procedure-related complications, communicating with the patient, health care team, patient's family, and referring physicians, and knowing who to call for help in case of problems. There should "be no surprises" in the intensive care setting, and the bronchoscopy/ICU team should be prepared for all eventualities, including but not limited to oxygen desaturation, hypotension, hypoxemia, dysrhythmias, agitation and anxiety, seizure, increased intracranial pressure, drug-related adverse events, copious difficult to remove secretions or mucous plugs, pneumothorax, bleeding, equipment malfunction, cardiac and respiratory arrest, and death.

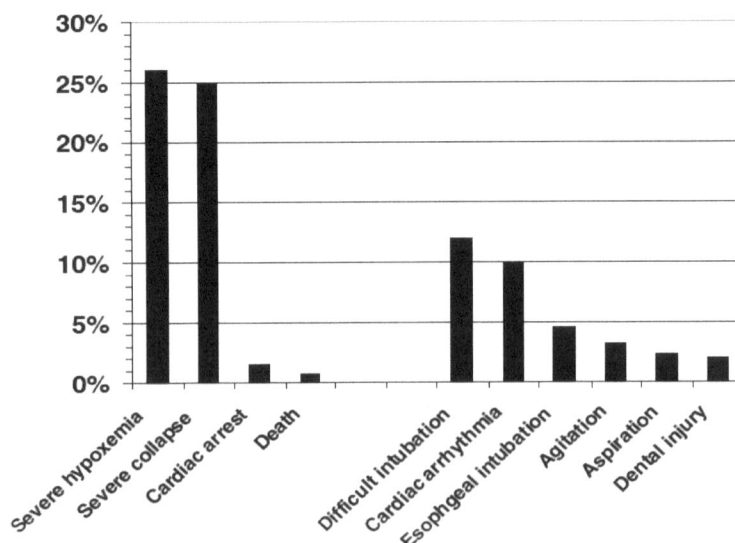

Graph reproduced from Jaber et al, Crit Care Med 2006;34:2355-2361.

References

1. Jaber S, Amraoui J, Lefrant Y et al. Clinical practice and risk factors for immediate complications of endotracheal intubation in the intensive care unit: a prospective multiple-center study. Crit Care Med 2006;34:2355-2361.

Question IV.22: Which of the following fruit represents an excellent mnemonic for remembering rules pertaining to the evaluation of the difficult airway?

A. APPLE
B. PEACH
C. LEMON

Answer IV.22   C

An excellent way to remember rules for evaluating the difficult airway is to remember the word LEMON, whereby the letters signify :

Look at the patient (examine for cachexia, scleroderma, flaccid tissues, facial abnormalities, trauma etc).
Evaluate 3-3-2-1 (3 fingers between upper and lower teeth (inter-incisor distance), 3 fingers between mentum and hyoid bone (thyromental distance), 2 fingers between thyroid notch and floor of the mandible (mandibulohyoid distance), 1 finger width of prognathia.
Mallampati class score.
Obstruction (such as tumors, avulsed teeth, burns, trauma, foreign bodies etc).
Neck mobility (usually decreased in the elderly. Examine for possible cervical spine fractures, rheumatoid arthritis, ankylosing spondylitis, neck brace, metastatic bone disease to the spine etc).

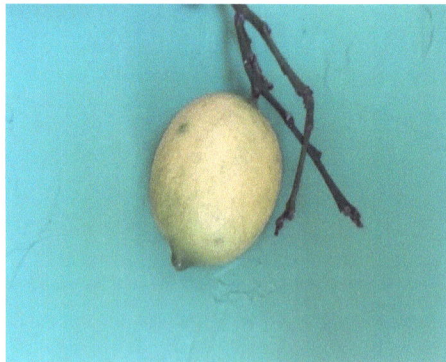

References

1. Boschert S. American College of Emergency Physicians News, November 2007. https://www.acep.org/content.aspx?id=33992#sm.00006v72z1dvxevhpbr1uuid7o2h1

Question IV.23:   The red arrow represents which component of the 3-3-2-1 score of a difficult airway evaluation?

A. The inter-incisor distance which should be at least 3 finger widths
B. The prognathia score which should be at least 1 finger width
C. The thyromental distance which should be at least 3 fingers widths
D. The mandibulohyoid distance which should be at least 2 finger widths

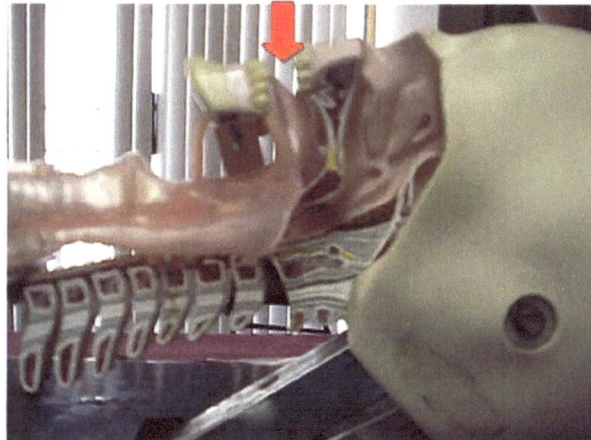

Answer IV.23:   A

The inter-incisor distance (between the upper and lower teeth) should be 3 finger widths. Overall, the 3-3-2-1 assessment represents an evaluation of the geometry of the oral, pharyngeal, and laryngeal axes, as well as the degree of prognathism which can make intubation more difficult. Other normal measurements are as follows:

- 3 fingers between mentum and hyoid bone (thyromental distance)
- 2 fingers between thyroid notch and floor of mandible (mandibulohyoid distance)
- 1 finger width of prognathia

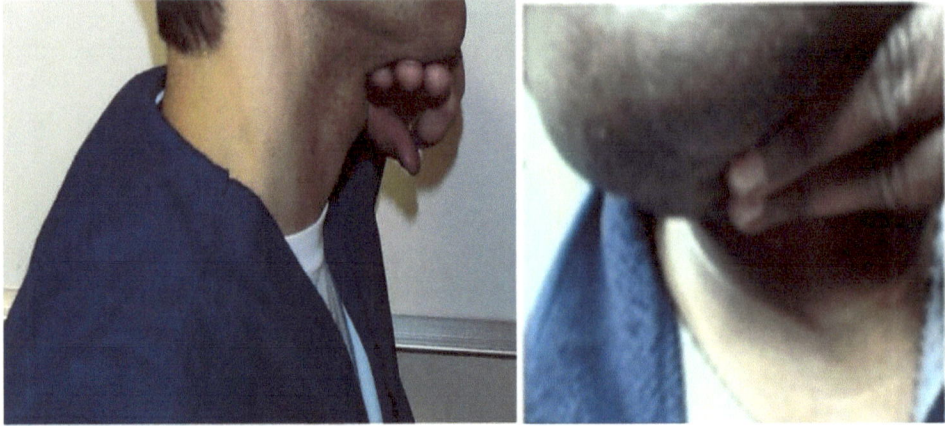

Thyromental (3 fingers) and mandibulohyoid (2 fingers) distances

Question IV.24: The Mallampati score of the patient represented in the Figure below is:

A. Class 1
B. Class 2
C. Class 3
D. Class 4

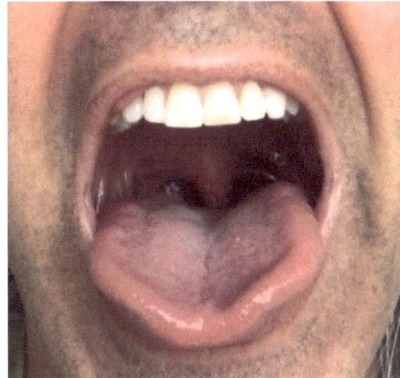

Answer IV:24:   B

This patient has a class 2 Mallampati score, which does not suggest a difficult airway. When checking the Mallampati score, patients should be examined sitting upright, with their head in a neutral position, mouth open and tongue maximally protruded (1). There is no need to as patients to say "ah".

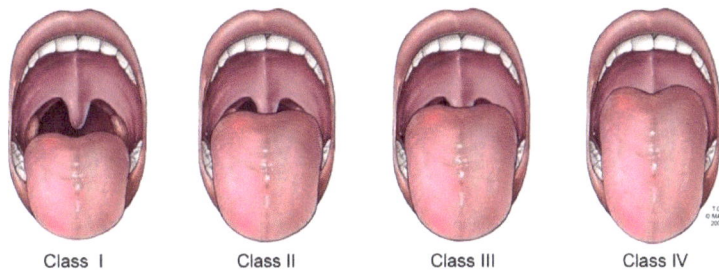

Class I   Class II   Class III   Class IV

References

1. Mallampati SR, et al. A clinical sign to predict difficult tracheal intubation: A prospective study. Can Anaesth Soc J. 1985; 32: 429-34.

Question IV.25: Why is the patient in the Figure below a potentially difficult airway?

A. Poor dentition, possible loose teeth, Mallampati score class 1, probably inter-incisor distance less than 2 finger widths.
B. Poor dentition, possible loose teeth, Mallampati score probably greater than 2, probably inter-incisor distance greater than 3 finger widths.
C. Poor dentition, possible loose teeth, large tongue, probably inter-incisor distance equal or less than 3 finger widths and Mallampati score probably greater than 2.

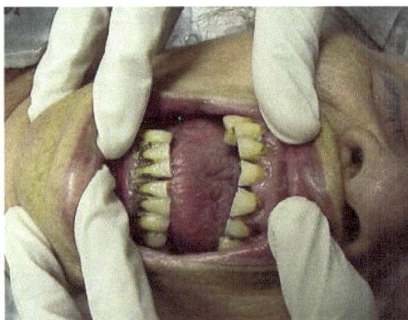

Answer IV.25:   C

This patient has obviously poor dentition and possible loose teeth. Each should be checked as necessary and of course, the patient should have been asked if he was awake and alert prior to the procedure. His tongue is obviously large and retracted in its relaxed state. Moderate sedation has perhaps already been administered, or the patient was unconscious prior to intubation. The inter-incisor distance certainly appears to be equal or less than 3 finger widths and the Mallampati score is probably greater than 2.

Question IV.26: The intubation-oral airway pictured below allows visualization of the larynx and vocal cords, even if the airway is inserted too far. This oral airway is called:

A. A Berman pharyngeal airway.
B. A Williams airway intubator.
C. An Ovassapian intubating airway.

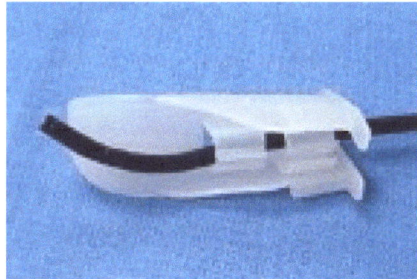

Answer IV.26:   C

Oral intubating airways help the bronchoscopist keep the flexible bronchoscope in the midline, expose laryngeal structures, and maintain an open pharynx. The Ovassapian fiberoptic intubating airway provides an open space in the oropharynx and protects the bronchoscope from being bitten by the patient. The airway can be removed without disconnecting the endotracheal tube adaptor. The wider distal half of the airway prevents the tongue and soft tissues of the anterior pharyngeal wall from falling back and obstructing the view of the glottis. The proximal half has a pair of guide walls that provide a space for the bronchoscope and endotracheal tube. This airway accommodates endotracheal tubes up to 9 mm inner diameter.

The Berman airway is also recommended for bronchoscopic intubation, but its length and tubular shape hinder maneuverability of the flexible bronchoscope once it is inserted. If the distal end of this airway is not perfectly in line with the glottic aperture, the airway must be partially withdrawn in order to expose the vocal cords.

The Williams airway intubator was designed for blind orotracheal intubation. Its distal half has an open lingual surface, which makes lateral and anteroposterior maneuverability of the bronchoscope difficult. In order to remove the Williams airway after intubation, the endotracheal tube adaptor must be removed prior to intubation.

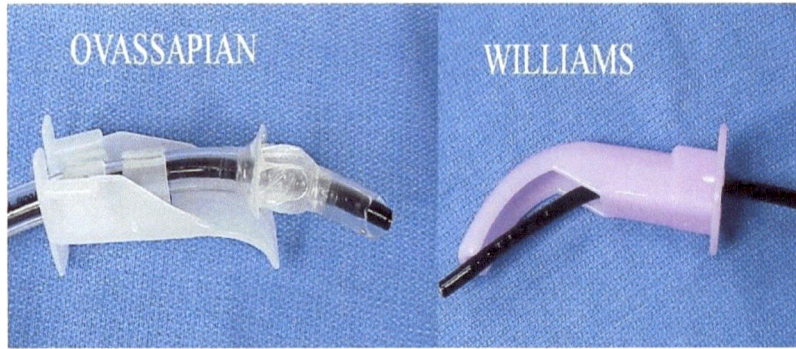

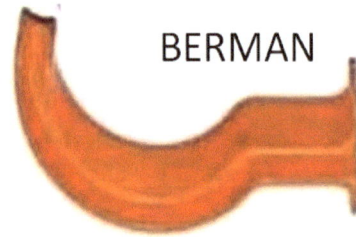

Examples of oral intubating airways

Question IV.27: A 37-year-old male with a history of high tracheal stenosis and metal stent insertion is emergently hospitalized in your intensive care unit. He has increasing tachypnea, cough, and hemoptysis. His oxygen saturation is 90 wearing 2 liters via nasal canula. He is using accessory muscles to breathe and appears extremely anxious. You perform flexible bronchoscopy without sedation because you suspect he may have a life-threatening recurrent subglottic stricture. Based on the finding in the Figure below, you elect to:

A. Perform an awake intubation using a #6 endotracheal tube over the bronchoscope inserted through the nares to rapidly secure an airway. You suspect the patient will require urgent rigid bronchoscopy with dilation and stent revision using rigid bronchoscopy and general anesthesia.
B. Proceed with rapid sequence intubation, and using a laryngoscope you attempt intubation using a #8 endotracheal tube in order to simultaneously dilate the stricture, tamponade the bleeding areas and assure the largest airway possible for ventilation.
C. You place an oral airway/bite block, increase oxygen flow via nasal canula, then proceed with moderate sedation, after placing the patient in the fully reclining position with a small pad under the head. Your plan is oral intubation with a #7.5 endotracheal tube over the flexible bronchoscope.

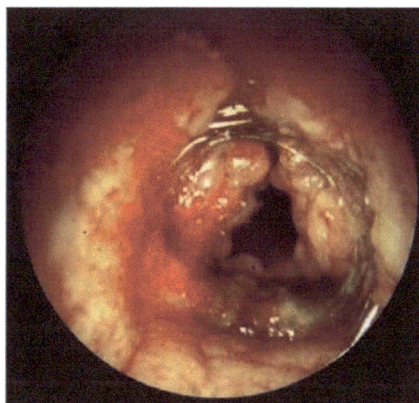

Answer IV.27:   A

The patient is in a life-threatening situation. The subglottic metal stent (a poor indication, and frequently a contraindication to metal stent placement) has partially ruptured and is ineffective at maintaining airway patency or palliating the stricture. Each of the proposed solutions has both risks and benefits. The best answer depends not only on the bronchoscopist's technical skill but also on personal biases and experience. While many would choose to first secure an airway by intubating with an uncuffed #6 tube, others would attempt using a cuffed tube despite the danger or metal struts puncturing the endotracheal tube balloon. Also, using a #6 endotracheal tube can be dangerous because the tube may be too short and not allow passage beyond the stenosis, especially for taller individuals. Others would prefer Rapid sequence intubation and intubation using a rigid laryngoscope, although the risk of permanently losing the airway is real and it may be necessary to use a tube smaller than a #8 tube. Any repeated failed attempts at intubation will cause mucosal swelling and more bleeding, with further loss of the airway, so the appropriate selection of a correct-sized endotracheal tube at the first attempt is essential. Placing the patient first in a sniff position, and sedating him can result in loss of the airway. It would be wiser to perform the intubation in a seated position, the bronchoscopist approaching the patient from the front. The bite block is essential to prevent damaging the bronchoscope that is introduced through the mouth.

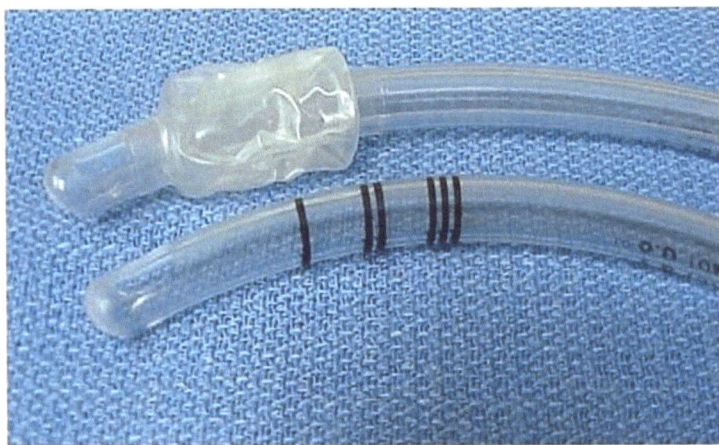

Cuffed and uncuffed #6 endotracheal tubes

References

1. Freitag L. Airway stents. Chapter 14. Interventional Pulmonology: European Respiratory Monograph. Strausz F and Bolliger CT Eds. Monograph 48, June 2010, pgs 197-216.
2. Davis N, Madden BP, Sheth A et al. Airway management of patients with tracheobronchial stents. British J Anesthesiol 2006;96:132-135.

Question IV.28: A forty-year-old patient is admitted to the intensive care unit for observation following complaints of increasing shortness of breath with exertion, hoarseness, and recurrent bouts of aspiration. There is a history of Lyme disease, but no history of stroke, thyroid surgery, cervical trauma, tuberculosis, cancer, or diphtheria. The chest radiograph is normal. Which of the following statements about unilateral vocal cord paralysis noted in the Figure below is correct?

A. About half of unilateral paralyzes are neoplastic in origin.
B. Lyme disease, as well as demyelinating diseases, neurotoxins such as arsenic and mercury, and viral neuronitis, are known causes of unilateral vocal cord paralysis.
C. Right vocal cord paralysis is more frequently encountered than left vocal cord paralysis.

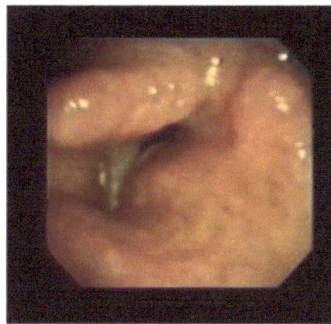

Answer IV.28:   B

This patient has unilateral right vocal cord paralysis. One-third of unilateral vocal cord paralyzes are neoplastic, one third are traumatic, and one third are idiopathic. Viral neuronitis is likely the most frequent cause of "idiopathic" vocal cord paralysis (1). The left vocal cord is paralyzed more frequently than the right, however, because the left recurrent nerve is longer than the right in its trajectory from the brainstem to the larynx, and thus more prone to injury from surgery, trauma, or compression.

References

1. Rosenthal LS. Etiology, incidence, and prevalence of laryngeal disorders. Chapter 34. From Sataloff's Comprehensive Textbook of Otolaryngology: Head and Neck Surgery. Sataloff RT and Benninger MS, Eds. Jaypee Brothers Medical Publishers, 2016.

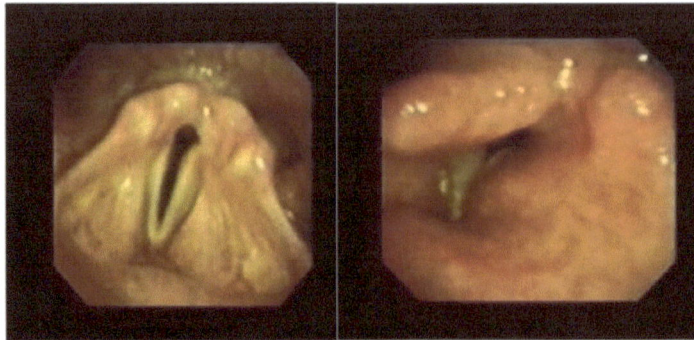

Normal vocal folds   Right vocal fold paralysis

References

1. Paquette CM et al. Unilateral vocal cord paralysis: a review of CT findings, mediastinal causes, and the course of the recurrent laryngeal nerves. Radiographics 2012;32(3), http://dx.doi.org/10.1148/rg.323115129

Question IV.29: An adult male with increasing hoarseness, deepening voice, dyspnea, and a history of severe gastroesophageal reflux is placed in the Intensive Care Unit overnight for observation. He smokes and occasionally uses cocaine. The following morning flexible bronchoscopy is performed. The Figure below is most consistent with:

A. Reinke's edema
B. Unilateral laryngeal cancer
C. Severe gastroesophageal reflux

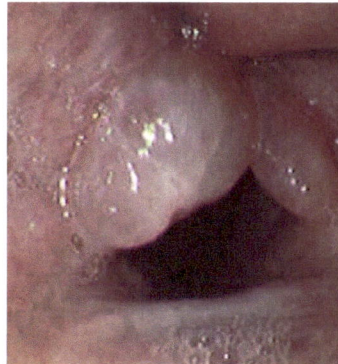

Answer IV.29:　　　A

　　　Reinke's edema is most prevalent in smokers with a history of gastroesophageal reflux. While it is sometimes bilateral, it can present as a swollen, gelatinous fluid filled Reinke space surrounding a vocal fold. It is a benign disorder and represents about 10 percent of benign laryngeal pathologies (1). Severe reflux can also cause laryngeal swelling, often with associated inflammation and chronic cough. Laryngeal cancers can have multiple different appearances from carcinoma in situ to large polypoid obstructing lesions. Consultation with an expert otorhinolaryngologist/ear, nose and throat surgeon is warranted. Speech and voice therapy consultations are often helpful. Close follow-up of laryngeal abnormalities is warranted because of possible malignant degeneration, risks of misdiagnosis, surveillance, and to assure response to therapy (2).

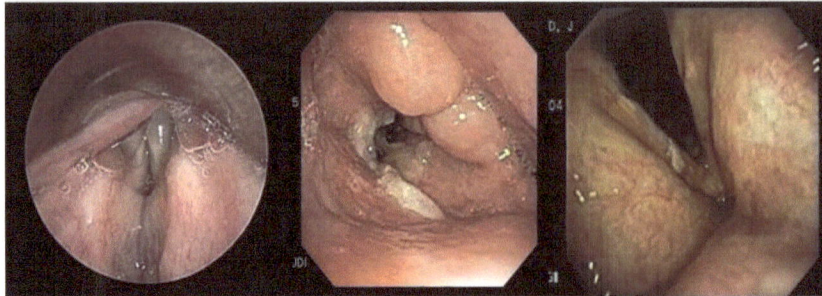

Laryngospasm at intubation   Laryngeal cancer/necrosis   Leukoplakia right vocal cord

References

1. Altman MD, Ph.D., Ken W. (2002). The Center for Voice, Northwestern University. Benign Vocal Lesions - Nodules, Polyps, Cysts.
2. Martins, Regina Helena Garcia (2009). "Is Reinke's Edema a Precancerous Lesion? Histological and Electron Microscopic Aspects". Journal of Voice. 23: 721–725. doi:10.1016/j.jvoice.2008.03.001.

Question IV.30: The bronchoscopic finding shown in the image below is seen in some patients with a history of cocaine use, chronic sinusitis, polyangiitis, or a chronic cough.

A. True
B. False

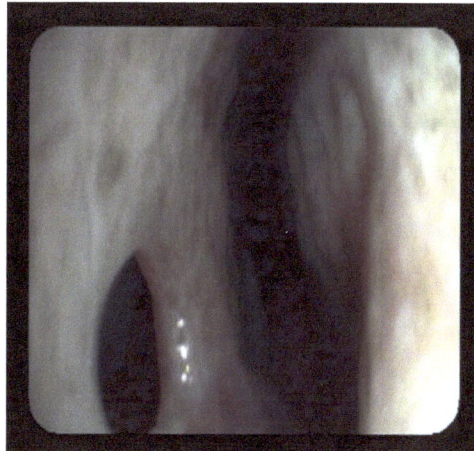

Answer IV.30:   A

The image shows a chronic, perforated nasal septum during bronchoscopy via the right nares. Causes include cocaine use, Granulomatous polyangiitis (GPA), other traumatic/iatrogenic nasal drug use, prolonged nasal intubation, exposure to toxic gases, and inflammatory and infectious diseases and neoplasms (1). While approximately two-thirds of people affected show no nasal complaints, others have chronic sinusitis, pain, or a chronic cough.

The most common cause of nasal septal perforation is an iatrogenic laceration of the mucoperichondrium bilaterally during a septoplasty. Diseases such as leishmaniasis, leprosy, GPA, sarcoidosis, rhinoscleroma, and syphilis, among others can also cause perforation. Traumatic events, such as chemical cauterization for epistaxis, and even chronic use of nasal corticosteroids and nasal vasoconstrictors are etiologic factors. GPA and sarcoidosis are the inflammatory diseases most commonly associated with septal perforation. Even disease affecting collagen and bone, such as systemic lupus erythematosus, can result in nasal perforation.

Whenever bronchoscopy is performed via the nares, physicians should carefully examine the upper airway anatomy (nares, septum, pharynx, and larynx) and be able to recognize both normal and abnormal findings.

References

1. Aurélio Fornazieri M Herrero Moreira J, Pilan R et al. Perforation of the nasal septum: etiology and diagnosis. International archives of otorhinolaryngology 2010:14(4);467-471.

***

CONGRATULATIONS

You have now completed Module IV of The Essential Intensivist Bronchoscopist©.

The following section contains a ten question post-test and answers.

Post-tests are True/False. Please remember that while many programs consider 70% correct responses a passing grade, the student's "target" score should be 100%.

Please send us your opinion regarding Bronchoscopy Education Project materials by contacting your national bronchology association or emailing us at www.bronchoscopy.org.

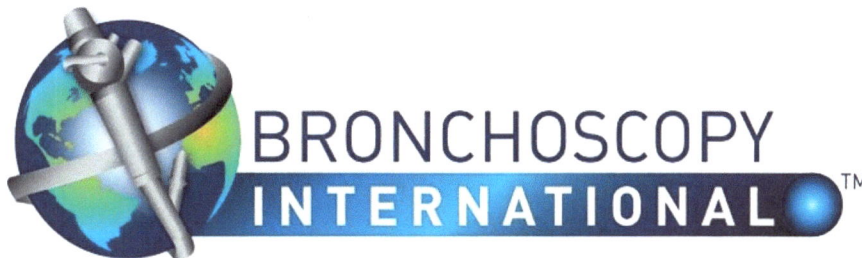

MODULE IV

TEN QUESTION TRUE/FALSE POST-TEST

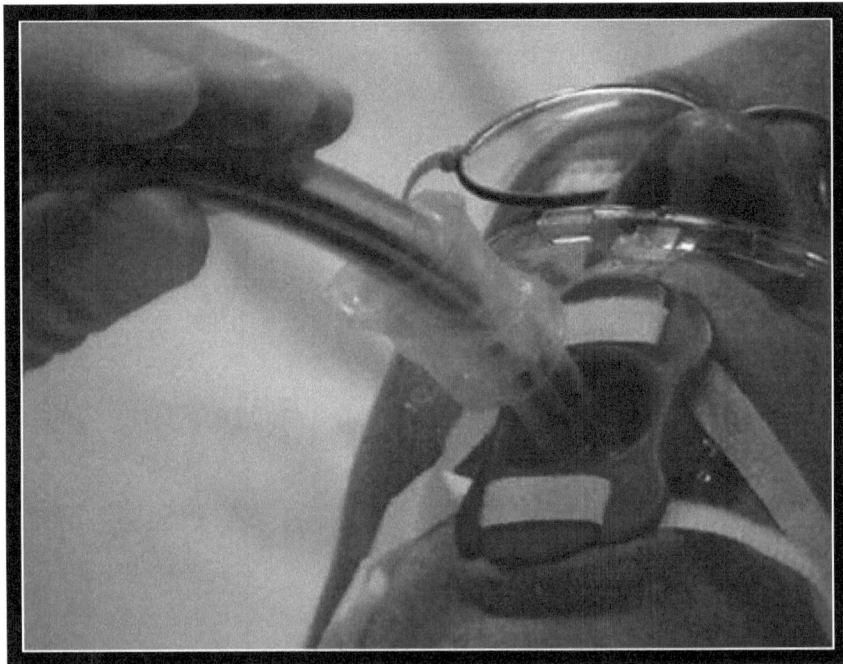

The Essential Intensivist Bronchoscopist

Module IV Post-test

INSTRUCTIONS: Answer True or False to each of the following <u>TEN</u> questions.

Question 1: In addition to its amnestic and hypotensive effects, Propofol provides analgesia.

Question 2: Difficulty to ventilate a patient after placement of an endobronchial blocker for hemoptysis may signal migration. Bronchoscopy is immediately warranted.

Question 3: Maximum upper airway edema may peak up to 48 hours after inhalation injury.

Question 4: Midazolam is the agent of choice for awake endotracheal intubation.

Question 5: Cardiac arrhythmias are a frequent complication of difficult airway management in the ICU.

Question 6: The uvula is not visible in patients with Mallampati score III.

Question 7: To avoid being « tongued out » during flexible bronchoscopy, a bite block should be secured and held firmly in place, even in sedated patients.

Question 8: Awake intubation is best performed with patients in the sitting position.

Question 9: A multidisciplinary team approach to difficult airway management is in the best interests of many critically ill patients.

Question 10: In critically ill patients, informed consent is often performed emergently, and therefore rarely requires a description of alternative procedures or a discussion of the consequences of not performing a certain procedure.

***

Answers to

The Essential Intensivist Bronchoscopist

post-test Module IV

ANSWERS

1. False
2. True
3. True
4. False
5. True
6. False
7. True
8. True
9. True
10. False

TOTAL SCORE _____/10

CONGRATULATIONS

You have now completed

The Essential Intensivist Bronchoscopist

This is an important achievement on your journey to competency. We know that you will use what you have learned to enhance your bronchoscopy skills.

This reading assignment is complementary to other components of the Bronchoscopy in the ICU curriculum, just one step closer to becoming a more technically skilled, competent and knowledgeable bronchoscopist.

We encourage you to attend national and international professional medical society meetings around the world so that you may share your experiences with your colleagues. We also urge you to explore the Bronchoscopy International website (www.bronchoscopy.org) for other learning materials, and to search instructional videos on the BronchOrg YouTube site. (See Video)

We look forward to receiving your comments regarding this and other components of The Bronchoscopy Education Project.

Please do not hesitate to contact your regional bronchology association, or email us at www.bronchoscopy.org.

Thank you for participating in The Bronchoscopy Education Project!

§

NOTES

CONTRIBUTORS

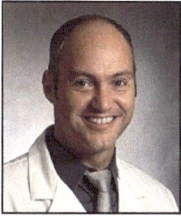

Dr. Septimiu Murgu is an Associate Professor of Pulmonary and Critical Care Medicine with the University of Chicago, and a certified Master Instructor with Bronchoscopy International. He has participated in Faculty Development programs in Singapore, Japan, India, Romania, and the United States. He is the coauthor of *The Essential EBUS Bronchoscopist* (Rake press), *The Essential cTBNA Bronchoscopist (Rake press)*, and of the best-selling medical textbook *Bronchoscopy and Central Airways Disorders: a patient-centered approach* (Elsevier press).

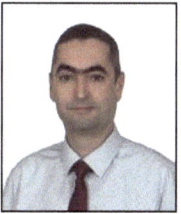

Dr. Tayfun Caliskan is an Assistant professor of pulmonary medicine in Sultan Abdulhamit Han Training and Research Hospital, Istanbul, Turkey. His interests include all aspects of interventional pulmonology. In addition to membership in the WABIP, Dr. Caliskan is a member of the Turkish Respiratory Society and of the European Respiratory Society.

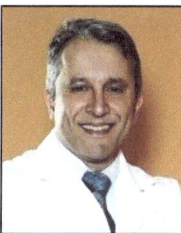

Dr. Hugo Goulart de Oliveira is Professor of Pulmonary Medicine, Universidade Federal do Rio Grande do Sul and Head of the Bronchoscopy Unit at the Hospital de Clínicas de Porto Alegre, Brazil. Dr. Oliveira is a Master Instructor with Bronchoscopy International/WABIP. His major interests include Interventional Pulmonology, and he is a recognized leader in endobronchial valve technology and its medical applications (particularly for patients with pneumothorax and emphysema).

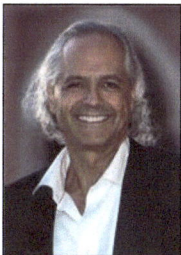

Henri Colt M.D. is Professor Emeritus at the University of California, an internationally recognized leadership coach, and award-winning medical educator. In addition to his leadership positions in professional medical societies, he conducts bronchoscopy, difficult airway management, and Train-the-Trainer instructional seminars around the world. His mission and that of his team of educators at Bronchoscopy International is to eliminate patient suffering caused by unequal physician expertise and inadequate on-the-job medical training. As a medical ethicist and expert in curricular design and competency-oriented processes, Dr. Colt provides consultative services to university faculty, governmental organizations, and national medical societies.

§

The **Essential Intensivist Bronchoscopist**© (EIB) is the fourth of six volumes in The Essential Bronchoscopist™ Series. It contains module-specific learning objectives, a series of ten-question true/false post-tests, and 120 question/answer sets pertaining to flexible bronchoscopy in the intensive care unit. Topics include indications and complications of bronchoscopy in critically ill patients, anesthesia and moderate sedation, percutaneous tracheostomy, bronchoscopy in mechanically ventilated patients, bronchoscopy using NIPPV, bronchoscopy in burn, inhalation, and traumatic injury victims, difficult airway management and bronchoscopic intubation, endobronchial valves for emphysema and pneumothorax, sampling strategies for patients with pulmonary infiltrates, bronchoscopy in central airway obstruction, and bronchoscopy in lung transplantation.

The aim of **The Essential Intensivist Bronchoscopist**© is to enrich the reader's knowledge of bronchoscopy in the intensive care unit and critical care setting. Question/answer sets can be used in low stakes knowledge assessments, interactive didactic slide presentations, and to promote conversation or debate with students, trainees, and colleagues. Detailed text, references, and figures help readers acquire cognitive knowledge, and illustrate many technical skills needed to become a competent bronchoscopist in the Intensive Care Unit and Critical Care setting.

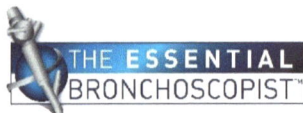

The Essential Bronchoscopist™ Series includes

- The Essential Flexible Bronchoscopist©
- The Essential cTBNA Bronchoscopist©
- The Essential EBUS Bronchoscopist©
- The Essential Intensivist Bronchoscopist©
- The Essential Interventional Bronchoscopist
- The Essentials of Bronchoscopy Education©

*The Essential Intensivist Bronchoscopist© is officially endorsed by professional medical associations and is a recommended reading assignment of the WABIP-endorsed Bronchoscopy Education Project.

THE ESSENTIAL BRONCHOSCOPIST© SERIES

Visit our website at:
www.bronchoscopy.org

THE ESSENTIAL INTENSIVIST BRONCHOSCOPIST©

rake
press

Laguna Beach, CA